New Aspects in Cesarean Sections

Edited by Panagiotis Tsikouras, Georg Friedrich Von Tempelhoff, Werner Rath and Nikolettos Nikos

Published in London, United Kingdom

New Aspects in Cesarean Sections
http://dx.doi.org/10.5772/intechopen.104332
Edited by Panagiotis Tsikouras, Georg Friedrich Von Tempelhoff, Werner Rath and Nikolettos Nikos

Contributors
Neha Sethi, Rajeev Kumar Rajaratnam, Nadiah Abdullah, Awol Yemane Legesse, Hale Teka, Salvatore Felis, Marta Fiamberti, Chiara Peluffo, Pablo Armas Cruz, Pablo Santillán Roldan, Andrés Cepeda Mora, Andres Sarmiento Benavides, Elisa Aucapiña Chocho, María Victoria Iturralde Arcos, Juan Carlos Jacome Sayay, María Isabel Jara Jimbo, Benjamin Joseph Nggada, Evangelia Antoniou, Eirini Orovou, Alexandros Papatrechas, Christiana Arampatzi, Panagiotis Eskitzis, Mulugeta W. Arage

First published in London, United Kingdom, 2023 by IntechOpen
IntechOpen is the global imprint of INTECHOPEN LIMITED, registered in England and Wales, registration number: 11086078, 5 Princes Gate Court, London, SW7 2QJ, United Kingdom

British Library Cataloguing-in-Publication Data
A catalogue record for this book is available from the British Library

Additional hard and PDF copies can be obtained from orders@intechopen.com

New Aspects in Cesarean Sections
Edited by Panagiotis Tsikouras, Georg Friedrich Von Tempelhoff, Werner Rath and Nikolettos Nikos
p. cm.
Print ISBN 978-1-83768-490-8
Online ISBN 978-1-83768-491-5
eBook (PDF) ISBN 978-1-83768-492-2

Meet the editors

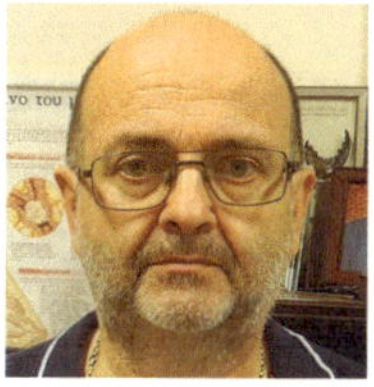

Panagiotis Tsikouras is a specialist in obstetrics and gynecology, perinatal medicine, and contraception at the School of Medicine, Democritus University of Thrace, Greece. He is also head of the Family Planning Centre and Gynecological Cytology Laboratory at the same university. Dr. Tsikouras is a fellow of the International Academy of Clinical and Applied Thrombosis/Hemostasis. His scientific activities focus on pediatric and adolescent medicine, gynecological oncology, and high-risk pregnancies. He is a reviewer for several international journals and has numerous scientific publications to his credit, including papers and book chapters. He has also contributed to international and national guidelines on coagulation and thrombosis in obstetrics and gynecology.

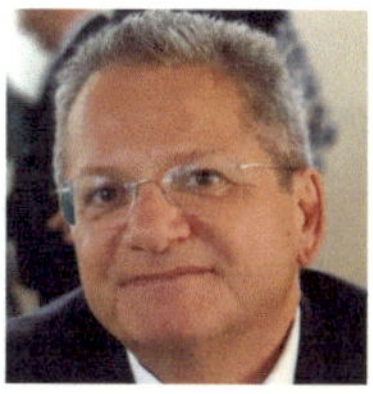

Prof. Nikolettos Nikos is a Professor of Obstetrics and Gynecology and Assisted Reproduction at the Democritus University of Thrace, Greece. He has training in gynecological endocrinology, human reproduction, and in vitro fertilization. From 2007 to 2011, he was the director of the In Vitro Fertilization Unit, University Regional General Hospital of Alexandroupolis, Greece. From 2012 to 2018, he was the director of the Laboratory of Reproductive Physiology-Artificial Fertilization. In 2019, he took over the management of the University Obstetrics-Gynecology Clinic of the Medical Department at the same university. His scientific work includes more than 100 publications in international journals and numerous invited lectures at international and Greek conferences.

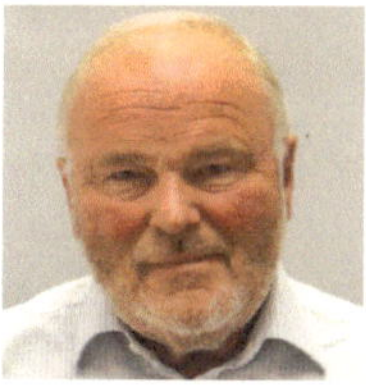

Prof. Dr. h. c. Werner Rath is a specialist in obstetrics and gynecology, gynecologic oncology, perinatal medicine, and hemostaseology. He was chief of the Department of Gynecology and Obstetrics, at University Hospital Aachen, Germany. He is a Professor of Gynecology and Obstetrics in the Faculty of Medicine, University Kiel, Germany. He received an Honorary doctorate from the University of Alexandroupolis. Dr. Rath is the recipient of several awards, including the Staude-Pfannenstiel Award of the North Germany Society of Gynecology and Obstetrics, the Maternité Award from the German Society of Perinatal Medicine, and the Berlin Harald-Bräutigam Award. His research and other activities include the Award of the Northern Society of Gynaecology & Obstetrics, Germany, and the Maternité Award from the German Society of Perinatal. His citable research publications are referred to since 1977. He is a reviewer for numerous journals.

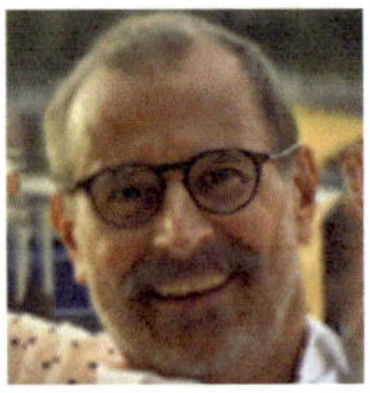

Prof. Dr. George Friedrich von Tempelhoff, FCATH, is a specialist in obstetrics and gynecology, gynecologic oncology, perinatal medicine, and hemostaseology. He is chief of the Department of Gynecology and Obstetrics, St. Vinzensius Hospital, Hanau Germany, and head of the Institute for Thrombosis and Coagulation Disorders in Gynecology and Obstetrics, Germany. He completed his medical education at Justus-Liebig University, Germany, and became a Consultant of Obstetrics and Gynecology in 1996. In 1993, he received his doctorate in medicine and completed his habilitation at the Johannes-Gutenberg University Mainz, Germany in 2007. He was appointed extracurricular professor at the Julius-Maximilians-Universität Würzburg, Germany in 2015. He is a fellow of the International Academy of Clinical and Applied Thrombosis/Hemostasis. His scientific focus is on hemostaseological and hemorheological disorders in women with miscarriages, preeclampsia, and thrombosis. Dr. Tempelhoff is a reviewer for numerous journals, author of several publications and book chapters, and a contributor to international and national guidelines on coagulation and thrombosis in gynecology.

Contents

Preface

At a global level, a great effort is being made to reduce the rates of cesarean sections (CS). The World Health Organization (WHO) defines "birth as a natural and normal function of life, which should not be approached as a disease." Vaginal labor is the benchmark, and CS should not exceed 15% of all births in a country. Per the WHO website: "Rather than recommending specific target rates, WHO underscores the importance of focusing on each woman's unique needs in pregnancy and childbirth In Europe, countries such as the Netherlands (CS rate of 15%) and Slovenia (CS rate of 14%) follow these standards.

According to recent studies, the continuous increase in the mean age of pregnant persons in developed countries and the simultaneous increase in multiple pregnancies due to in vitro fertilization (IVF) may have led to an increased percentage of CS estimated at about 30%. Worldwide, the frequency of CS has increased during the last 30 years. In the United States, the percentage of CS is around 32%. Greece has one of the highest percentages of CSs in Europe at 38% although there are no clear statistics that include all births. The percentage of CS is steadily increasing In Greece, 38% of children are born even though this operation should be applied only in special cases when the health of the child or mother is in danger. CS was not a common obstetric surgery 40 years ago, at which time its frequency was about 10%.

In the last decades, there was a dramatic increase in the frequency of CS (> 1%/ year). In the United States in 1986, CS rates approached the highest levels of about 25%. Since then, it has stabilized at around 22%. At the start of the 21st century, a new increase was observed with a frequency reaching 31.1% in 2006. In most European countries the percentage also exceeds 30%. The medical effects of this phenomenon remain unclear. This phenomenon is also observed in the developing countries of Latin America. For example, in Brazil the frequency of CS increased from 15% in 1970 to 43% in 2005.

Some possible reasons for the increased rate of CS include:

- improved technical performance combined with increased security
- reduction of maternal mortality
- increased frequency of pregnancy among persons older than 35 years
- firstborns with single pregnancies with head projection and with automatic or induced initiation of labor
- increased obstetric care (mass application of methods of monitoring the placental unit)

- increased medical fees (the price for CS is higher than for vaginal childbirth which potentially increases the profit margin)
- history of previous CS

Nowadays, there is a tendency for people to have fewer children, which has led to a greater proportion of firstborns who are known to be at high risk for CS. In addition, increased rates of twin (35%) and multiple (77%) pregnancies worldwide due to assisted reproduction measures have consequently increased rates of CS with sciatic projection. Other factors include the small stature of the pregnant person, which is associated with a 40% increased risk of CS, and pre-existing obesity in the pregnant person, which is associated with a 60% increased risk of CS. The above risk (body weight in pregnancy) does not include the increased birth weight or the increased incidence of diabetes and hypertension in the pregnant population. A forecasted newborn birth weight > 4000 gm is also associated with a threefold increase in the risk for CS. Pregnant persons have 40% increased rates of CS due to more frequent problems of dystocia (because of heavier weight) and fetal distress (the cause is unclear).

Indications for CS include a threat to the life of the mother or child and preventive signs by the mother or fetus health problems. Contraindications to CS include when the risk of surgery is greater than the risk to the fetus (hydrocephalus, extreme prematurity, stillbirth).

According to meta-analyses, the use of cardiotocographic monitoring of the placental unit led to an increase of 20% in the frequency of CS. This may be due to an overestimation of the records regarding the presence or absence of perinatal asphyxia. Several blind studies in which it has been reported that comparing CS after induction or waiting in pregnancy extension without fully documented conclusions and without significant differences. The method of active childbirth is applied mainly with the aim of reducing CS. However, the application of epidural analgesia is likely to increase in frequency (13% vs. 8% in the United States).

The increased frequency of primary CS led to an increase in the pool of pregnant persons with previous CS despite the last small increase in the rate of vaginal delivery after cesarean section. Regarding maternity hospitals, there are public and private maternity centers with high CS rates. In contrast, academic hospitals have lower rates even though they treat more high-risk pregnancies. This is due to their educational nature. Of particular interest are pregnancies in adolescents. According to researchers, 50% of births in adolescence have complications, resulting in a rate of CS approaching 27% for single pregnancies with head projection. The increased risk of prematurity and delayed intrauterine growth observed at these ages also contribute to the increase in CS rates.

Despite the relative safety of CS, it is accompanied by increased maternal morbidity and treatment costs. Therefore, efforts should be made to develop frequency reduction strategies. This requires increased attention and improved timely certification and treatment of problems that arise during childbirth. Particular attention should be paid to reducing the frequency of CS in firstborns with single pregnancy and head projection.

Panagiotis Tsikouras and Nikolettos Nikos
Professor,
Greece Department of Obstetrics and Gynecology,
Democritus University of Thrace,
Alexandroupolis, Greece

Georg Friedrich Von Tempelhoff
Department of Gynecology and Obstetrics,
St. Vinzenz Hospital Hanau,
Hanau, Germany

Werner Rath
Gynecology and Obstetrics Department,
Faculty of Medicine,
University Kiel,
Kiel, Germany

Section 1

Cesarean Section after Uterine Surgery and Vaginal Birth after Cesarean Section

Chapter 1

Labor Induction

Mulugeta W. Arage

Abstract

Introduction: Induction of labor is the process of artificially stimulating uterine contraction after the fetus has reached viability and before the spontaneous onset of labor for accomplishing vaginal delivery. It is a common obstetric procedure that is primarily indicated in the presence of complications that put continuing of pregnancy at risk. Its global rate is around 20% with great variation across regions. The most common indications are: postterm pregnancy, hypertensive disorders during pregnancy, pre-labor rupture of membrane, intrauterine growth restriction, intrauterine fetal death, abruption placenta, fetal congenital anomalies, and other medical disorders. Despite its huge significance in preventing neonatal and maternal mortality and morbidity, induction of labor by itself has its own risks and complications compared to spontaneous labor, including a potential of failure to progress, leading to cesarean birth and its complications. When deciding undertaking induction of labor and after fulfilling the requirements for induction, the next step will be deciding which methods will be used to achieve it. Induction could be done medically, surgically, or both depending on the indication and other conditions.

Keywords: labor induction, induction outcome, methods of induction, failed induction, oxytocin

1. Introduction

Labor induction is the stimulation of uterine contraction artificially after the fetus has reached viability (after the 28th week of gestation) and before the spontaneous onset of labor for accomplishing vaginal delivery [1]. It is a common obstetric procedure primarily employed in the presence of obstetrics and medical conditions that threaten pregnancy continuation [2, 3]. Induction of labor has its indications that could be can be elective (planned) or emergency. Elective induction is usually done with prior planning by the health- provider and the mother when continuing the pregnancy beyond certain weeks has risk for the mother or the fetus, like in the case of PROM, DM, moderate hypertension postdate pregnancy, small or large for date baby. Emergency induction is done when there is an emergency maternal and fetal condition that necessities induction of labor immediately such as prolonged PROM, severe IUGR, intrauterine infection, pregnancy beyond 42 week, and preeclampsia and eclampsia [4].

Unfortunately, despite its undisputed importance for ending risky pregnancy, compared with the spontaneous onset of labor, induction has a potential risk of increased rate of cesarean birth and its complication along with different maternal and neonatal complications [5, 6]. Due to this, the World Health Organization (WHO) recommends induction to be performed only with a clear medical indication when expected benefits outweigh potential harms [2].

Although oxytocin is an effective means of labor induction, in women with a favorable cervix, as noted earlier, it is less effective as a cervical ripening agent. Many RCTs that have compared oxytocin with various prostaglandin (PG) formulations and other methods of cervical ripening confirm this observation.

2. Prevalence

Nowadays, the prevalence of induction of labor in the field of obstetrics is increasing. According to a WHO report, up to 25% of all term deliveries in developed countries were following labor induction for different reasons. In the United States and England, labor induction accounts for 29% [4] of deliveries, while 12.1% and 4.4% of deliveries are induced in Asian and African regions, respectively [5].

However, even if induction of labor is practiced widely in the field of obstetrics, it has variations from setting to setting, with studies showing that facilities in developing countries tend to have lower rates of induction of labor than in developed countries. One systematic study shows that the average induction rate was 4.4% in African, 12.1% in Asian, and 11.4% in Latin American countries, which has a huge difference from that in developed countries [5, 6].

3. Indications and contraindications of induction of labor

The decision to induce labor was never an easy task and requires a complex clinical judgment. It usually constitutes a choice between three options, allowing the pregnancy to continue, inducing labor, or performing cesarean section, and needs the consideration of a number of factors [2]. Some of the factors are the condition of the baby, gestational age and the level of certainty about the baby's age (rarely, preterm induction may have to be done.), history of previous cesarean section, the preference of the mother, and the likelihood that induction of labor will be efficient and vaginal delivery could be achieved, which in turn is dependent on the state of the uterine cervix and birth canal [3, 7].

Taking the above conditions in to consideration, there are various indications that might require labor induction. These factors could be maternal or fetal and sometimes both.

3.1 Maternal indications

Maternal conditions that necessitate labor induction could be medical conditions or discomforts that have been caused or aggravated by pregnancy [8, 9]. These indications include:

- Preeclampsia/eclampsia

- Gestational hypertension ≥38 weeks
- Diabetes mellitus
- Renal disease
- Chronic pulmonary disease
- Cholestasis of pregnancy
- Abruptio placentae

3.2 Fetal indications

- Prolonged pregnancy
- Suboptimal intrauterine growth
- Chorioamnionitis
- Multiple pregnancy
- Polyhydramnios
- Uncomplicated twin pregnancy ≥38 weeks
- Pre-labor ruptured membranes
- Alloimmune disease at or near term
- Oligohydramnios
- Nonreassuring antepartum fetal testing
- Intrauterine fetal death

In addition to the abovementioned maternal and fetal indications, labor induction can be done for allowing the essential treatment to be commenced, such as for cervical cancer, relieving emotional distress after intrauterine death in previous pregnancy, or alleviating anxiety about the baby's well-being [10]. Likewise, although currently available guidelines do not recommend it, induction of labor is being used more and more at the request of pregnant women to shorten the duration of pregnancy or to time the birth of the baby according to the convenience of the mother and/or health-care workers [3, 5, 11, 12].

In general, the reason for induction varies from area to area. According to a study done in Latin America, premature rupture of membranes was the single most frequent medical indication accounting for 25.3% of the indications, while post-term pregnancy was the second most common. Another systematic study done in Africa shows that PROM was the most common (27.3%) reason for artificial initiation of labor [2]. In another study done in Saudi Arabia, the most common indication for IOL was post-term pregnancy accounting for (31%) cases followed by gestational and preexisting diabetes mellitus, together 23.2%, while PROM was the third most common indication accounting for 15% [12].

In conclusion, induction of labor is recommended when the risk of continuation of pregnancy either to the mother or to the fetus is more than that of continuing the pregnancy. However, sometimes induction for maternal interest may compel ignoring the fetus.

3.3 Unacceptable indications

- Care provider or patient convenience
- Impending macrosomia
- Patients considered to be at an increased risk for preeclampsia (such as having a prior history of preeclampsia)
- Concerns about intrauterine growth restriction
- Additionally, preterm or early-term induction is not medically indicated for maternal anxiety or discomfort related to normal pregnancy
- Previous pregnancy with labor abnormalities such as rapid labor or shoulder dystocia
- Simply because the mother lives far from the hospital
- Suspected fetal macrosomia (estimated fetal weight > 4000 gm) in a nondiabetic women is also an unacceptable indication because there is no reduction in the incidence of shoulder dystocia but twice the risk of CS [13, 14].

3.4 Contraindications

Induction should be avoided if there is any fetal or maternal condition that contraindicates labor or vaginal delivery. These conditions could be grouped as absolute and relative contraindications.

3.4.1 Absolute contraindications

Absolute contraindicates are any gynecological, obstetrical, or medical conditions that preclude safe vaginal delivery, which include but are not limited to the following [3, 15, 16]:

- Cephalopelvic disproportion more than borderline (macrosomia or contracted pelvis)
- Abnormal fetal lie or presentation (e.g., transverse or oblique lie, footling breech)
- Diagnosed major placenta or vasa previa

- Extensive vaginal plastic operations like repaired fistulas.
- Pelvic tumors obstructing delivery like cervical cancer and tumor previa
- Pelvic structural deformities
- Umbilical cord presentation and prolapse
- Abnormal fetal heart rate pattern (Category III fetal heart rate tracing)
- Absence of cesarean section facility
- Extensive genital wart, cervical cancer, and active genital herpes
- Previous history of uterine surgery like classical cesarean section or inverted T uterine incision, two or more lower segment cesarean sections, myomectomy entering the endometrial cavity, ruptured uterus, and so on.

3.4.2 Relative contraindications

- Elderly primigravida or grand multiparty
- Uterine over distention from polyhydramnios or multiple pregnancy
- One lower segment cesarean section
- Frank breech
- Bad obstetric history
- Unfavorable cervix, especially for elective induction.

N.B. These conditions require internal or external continuous monitoring of uterine contractions and the fetal heartbeat. In the absence of such monitoring, they become absolute contraindications [17].

4. Outcome of labor induction

Induction of labor (IOL) is done with the main aim of initiating labor without its true time to save the health of the mother and unborn fetus and minimizing severe obstetric complications related to unnecessary cesarean section [2]. However, this artificial initiation of labor is not without its own risks and is associated with adverse maternal and perinatal outcomes such as postpartum hemorrhage [18], hyperstimulation of the uterus that can result in uterine rupture, chorioamnionitis, endometritis [9], fetal hypoxia, maternal fluid intoxication [19], stillbirth [5], severe birth asphyxia [20], increased medical interventions, increased hospital costs [3], abnormal fetal heart rate patterns, maternal water intoxication if oxytocin is used, delivery of a preterm infant due to incorrect estimation of dates, and cord prolapse [8, 21]. Induction of labor also influences the woman's childbirth experience, and it has more discomfort and pain. For these abovementioned reasons before starting IOL, all pregnant women should have consented to the process and understand all benefits, maternal and fetal risks, and alternatives to IOL. Furthermore, reviewing indications for cesarean section, operative vaginal delivery should be discussed prior to offering IOL.

Furthermore, even after induction is done knowing all these risks, it might not achieve the intended labor and vaginal birth, and it may result in failed induction. However, while there is a well-accepted definition of IOL, the definition of a successful or failed induction of labor (FIOL) is less certain [22–24]. Most studies define FIOL as an inability to achieve vaginal delivery or birth through cesarean section (CS) [25–27]. Nevertheless, others suggest a variety of criteria such as mode of delivery (vaginal versus cesarean) and certain time intervals within which active phase of labor is achieved or adequate number of uterine contractions is achieved for diagnosing FIOL [3, 28, 29]. Some protocols also define it as failure to achieve regular (e.g., every 3 min) uterine contractions and cervical change after at least 6–8 h of the maintenance dose of oxytocin administration, with artificial rupture of membranes [30]. American College of Obstetricians and Gynecologists (ACOG) recommends diagnosing and doing cesarean section for a failed IOL if vaginal delivery is not achieved for 12–18 hours after administrating oxytocin and performing amniotomy [16].

5. Pre-induction assessment

As mentioned before, although the goal of labor induction is to achieve a successful vaginal delivery, induction exposes women to a higher risk of a CS and other complications than spontaneous labor. To minimize these risks and complications, thorough examination of the maternal and fetal condition is required before undertaking labor induction [31]. Indications and contraindications for induction should be well reviewed and discussed with the patient along with the alternatives, risks, and benefits of labor induction. Confirmation of gestational age and evaluation of fetal lung maturity should also be performed. Labor induction should be performed at a location where personnel who are familiar with the process and its potential complications are available. Availability of uterine activity and electronic fetal monitoring (EFM) is also recommended for any mothers receiving uterotonic medications [2, 32].

In spite of this, existing evidence points out that the failure rate of IOL is increasing worldwide [33, 34]. As a result, a variety of maternal and fetal factors as well as screening tests have been suggested to predict labor induction success. Maternal factors include: parity (prior vaginal delivery), body mass index (BMI), and maternal age. Fetal factors include: estimated fetal weight, gestational age, and fetal presentation. Clinical pelvimetry, transvaginal ultrasound (TVUS) assessment of the cervix, and biochemical markers [including fetal fibronectin (fFN) and insulin-like growth factor binding protein-1 (IGFBP-1) [31, 35, 36]]. The other main factor that determines the success of induction is the status of the cervix (Bishop score) before induction is commenced. For this reason, before undertaking induction of labor, pre-induction assessment for the fulfillment of the prerequisites, particularly bishop score, is required.

5.1 Cervical ripening and Bishop score

One of the main factor that needs to be examined and documented before labor induction is cervical status using Bishop score, which is one of the most important factors for predicting the likelihood of success in labor induction [31, 37]. The Bishop score is a pre-labor pelvic scoring system that is commonly used in clinical practice as a predictor of the success for induction [38].

It was first developed in the 1960s by Dr. Edward Bishop. Initially, the system tabulates a score based on 5 determinants (the station of the presenting part and four characteristics of the cervix) [39]:

1. Dilation,
2. Effacement,
3. Consistency, and
4. Position.

Each component attributes a value from 0 to 2 or 3 points each (for a maximum score of 13). However, in 1966, Burnett modified the scoring scheme so that each variable was assigned a maximum value of 2 points (for a maximum score of 10) [40].

If the Bishop score is high, which is often considered to be a score of 8 or above, the likelihood of vaginal delivery is similar whether labor is spontaneous or induced [41]. In contrast, a low Bishop score, which is a score of 5 or less, is considered to be unfavorable, and if an induction is indicated, cervical ripening agents may be utilized [37, 38, 41]. A score from 6 to 7 is considered to be intermediate [30, 32].

Several studies have shown an increased rate of failed induction and CS when women are induced with an unfavorable cervix (12–16). Xenakis's prospective study of 597 pregnancies stratified found the highest risk of CS and failed induction in those with low Bishop scores [25].

6. Method of induction and cervical ripening

When deciding undertaking induction of labor after fulfilling the requirements for induction, the next step will be deciding which methods will be used to achieve it. Depending on different conditions, there are different types of induction methods that could be utilized. These methods are grouped as medical and surgical. Medical method of induction are methods that use pharmacological products to achieve artificial labor initiation, while surgical methods use non-pharmacological methods [2, 3, 31, 32].

6.1 Medical method

6.1.1 Prostaglandins

Prostaglandins are a group of physiologically active endogenous compounds found in the myometrium, decidua, and fetal membranes during pregnancy. Its administration results in the dissolution of collagen bundles and an increase in submucosal water content of the cervix, resulting in changes of cervical connective tissue that are similar to those observed in early labor [2, 3, 31, 42]. It also causes direct stimulation of myometrial contraction by stimulating receptors in the uterus [38].

PG formulations analogues were have been used since they were first synthesized in the laboratory in 1968. They could be used for both induction and as a cervical ripening agent, but they are more effective when used for cervical ripening with increased success of vaginal delivery rates within 24. However, the overall risk of cesarean section will not change, and they have an increased risk of uterine hyperstimulation and FHR changes [43].

Although they can be given intravenously and by oral routes, local administration of PGs in the vagina or the endocervix is the route of choice because of fewer side effects and acceptable clinical response [31].

There are different types and preparations of PG available for both induction of labor and cervical ripening.

Prostaglandin E2 (PGE2): Also known by the name dinoprostone, it is a naturally occurring compound involved in promoting labor, by causing contractions in the myometrium via direct stimulation and softening and dilatation in the cervix, dissolving the collagen structural network of the cervix [38, 42].

Prostaglandin E2 is available in 3 different preparations as a cervical ripening agent:

- Intravaginal 1 mg and 2 mg gel (Prostin), and

A. **Intravaginal Cervidil**

- It is a vaginal insert form of PGE2 that contains 10 mg of dinoprostone in a timed-release formulation.
- It releases the medication at 0.3 mg/hr. that could be left in place for up to 12 hours, and oxytocin may be initiated from 30 to 60 minutes after its removal [31].

B. **Intracervical gel (Prepidil) [31].**

- It contains dinoprostone, 0.5 mg per 3 g syringe (2.5 mL gel), for intracervical administration.
- Its dose can be repeated in 6–12 hours if cervical change is inadequate and uterine activity is minimal following the first dose. However, drug administration should cease if there are no contractions within twenty-four hours or if there are severe adverse effects, including membrane rupture or uterine hyperstimulation [32, 44].
- The recommended maximum cumulative dose of dinoprostone should not exceed 1.5 mg (three doses) within a 24-hour period.
- Because of the potential for uterine tachsystole with concurrent oxytocin and prostaglandin administration, oxytocin should not be initiated until 6–12 hours after the last dose of dinoprostone [44].

C. **Intravaginal gel (Prostin),**

- It is a translucent triacetin-based thixotropic gel formulation that contains either 1 mg or 2 mg of dinoprostone, as the active ingredient in each unit dose of 3 grams (2.5 mL).

- It is inserted high into the posterior fornix of the vagina, and patient should be instructed to remain recumbent for at least 30 minutes.

- For women with favorable cervix, the initial dose is 1 mg of PROSTIN E2 Vaginal Gel.

The advantage of the controlled-release vaginal insert (Cervidil) over the intracervical one is that it easier to administrate than intracervical (Prepidil) preparations, and it allows easier removal in the case of onset of active labor, rupture of membranes, or with the development of uterine tachsystole. It also requires only a 30 minute delay before the initiation of oxytocin upon its removal compared with an interval of 6 hours for the latter [32, 42].

In conclusion, as other methods, the use of PGE2 has its own advantages and limitations.

Advantages:

- Good patient acceptance,
- A lower operative rate than oxytocin and less need for oxytocin augmentation when used with an unfavorable cervix (Bishop <7) [32]
- It is a bronchodilator and is not contraindicated in women who suffer from asthma.

Limitations:

- Relatively expensive,
- Requires refrigerated storage and is unstable at room temperature,
- Has more chorioamnionitis or endometritis and admissions to NICU than oxytocin [31].

Prostaglandin E1 (Misoprostol): It is another form of synthetic prostaglandine1 analogue that has uterotonic properties, by contracting smooth muscle fibers in the myometrium and facilitation of cervical opening by relaxing of the cervix [45]. It is considered as a safe and effective off-label use for induction of labor or cervical ripening by ACOG [46]. It is available as 100 μg and 200 μg tablets that could be divided to provide 25 or 50 μg doses.

Due to higher dosing (50 μg every 6 hours), it may be associated with uterine tachsystole and fetal heart rate decelerations; ACOG recommends using 25 μg dosing every 3–6 hours with vaginally applied misoprostol and suggests that the higher doses should be used only in select circumstances [47]. If necessary, oxytocin may be initiated 4 hours after the final misoprostol dose in using 25 μg.

A meta-analysis that compared 25 μg with 50 μg dosing reported that 50 μg dosing resulted in a higher rate of vaginal delivery within 24 hours with higher rates of uterine tachsystole meconium passage and higher frequency of fetal acidosis with an umbilical arterial pH of less than 7.16 but without compromising the neonatal outcomes [48].

Advantages of misoprostol are that it is inexpensive, stable at room temperature, and can be administered orally or placed vaginally with few systemic side effects. However, compared with vaginal misoprostol, administration of misoprostol by the buccal or sublingual route increases uterine tachsystole [31].

Mode of administration: Misoprostol can be administered orally or placed vaginally with few systemic side effects, with studies reporting that misoprostol tablets placed vaginally are either superior to or equivalent in efficacy compared with intracervical PGE2 gel [49]. Although no difference in clinical outcomes are apparent when comparing intravaginal or intracervical PGE2 preparations, for ease of administration and patient satisfaction, vaginal administration is recommended [48, 50, 51].

NOTE: PG formulations of any kind should be avoided in women with a prior uterine scar, such as a prior cesarean delivery or myomectomy, because their use has been associated with an increased risk of uterine rupture.

6.1.2 Oxytocin

Oxytocin is the most potent uterotonic and common pharmacologic agent used to induce labor. It stimulates the smooth muscles of the uterus in similar fashion with the natural hormone that secretes from the posterior lobe of the pituitary gland in a pulsatile fashion. It also causes contraction of the myoepithelial cells surrounding the mammary alveoli leading to milk ejection during lactation [31, 52].

It has been used either alone or with other drugs and methods. Its administration produces periodic uterine contractions first demonstrable at approximately 20 weeks' gestation, with increasing responsiveness with advancing gestational age primarily due to the upregulation of oxytocin receptor MRNA levels and strong increase in the density of myometrial oxytocin receptors, reaching a peak during early labor [31, 53]. **Once spontaneous labor begins, the uterine sensitivity to oxytocin increases rapidly.** This physiologic mechanism makes oxytocin less effective as a cervical ripening agent [31].

Although oxytocin is an effective means of labor induction, in women with a favorable cervix, as noted earlier, it is less effective as a cervical ripening agent and commonly used in combination with other cervical ripening methods. It could also be used alone given the cervix is favorable [54].

Oxytocin protocols and mode of administration: Oxytocin is most often given intravenously and cannot be given orally because the polypeptide could be degraded to small, inactive forms by gastrointestinal enzymes. Its plasma half-life is short, estimated at 3–6 minutes, and steady-state concentrations are reached within 30–40 minutes of initiation or dose change.

It is generally diluted by placing 10 units in 1000 mL of an isotonic solution, such as normal saline, yielding an oxytocin concentration of 10 mU/mL. And given by infusion pump to allow continuous, precise control of the dose is administered [31, 32]. The dosage can be divided into high-dose and low-dose protocols depending on the initial dose and the amount and rate of sequential increase in dose [47, 52].

However, despite the frequent use of oxytocin in clinical practice, and suggestion of several experts for the implementation of a standardized protocol in oxytocin administration [47, 55]. There is little consensus regarding which protocol is most appropriate. And oxytocin protocols in induction of labor remain one of the challenges in the field of obstetrics. Protocols differ as to the initial dose, incremental time period, and steady-state dose [47].

Low-dose oxytocin protocols

- They mimic endogenous maternal physiology and are associated with lower rates of uterine tachsystole
- They are initiated at 0.5–1 mU and increased by 1 mU/min at 30- to 40-minute intervals.
- An alternative low dose begins at 1 to 2 mU/min that is increased by 2 mU/ min with shorter incremental time intervals of 15–30 minutes.

High-dose oxytocin protocols

- They often start with an initial oxytocin dose of 6 mU/min that is increased by 6 mU/min at 15- to 40-minute intervals or start at 4 mU/ min with 4 mU/min incremental increases every 15 minutes [31, 56].
- A maximum oxytocin dose has not been established, but most protocols do not exceed 42 mU/min [31].
- These regimens are largely used in active management of labor protocols and for labor augmentation, rather than for labor induction.

6.2 Mechanical and surgical methods

6.2.1 Stripping or sweeping of the fetal membranes

Stripping or sweeping of the fetal membranes refers to the digital separation of the chorioamniotic membrane from the wall of the cervix and lower uterine segment by inserting the examiner's finger beyond the internal cervical os and then rotating the finger circumferentially along the lower uterine segment [31]. Sweeping of the membranes is simple, safe procedure and could be used as both labor induction and cervix ripening method. It is thought to cause ripening of the cervix and eventually labor by inducing the release of endogenous prostaglandins from the membranes and decidua. It also triggers Ferguson reflex, which promotes oxytocin release from maternal pituitary. It is usually done prior to ARM as a preliminary step or could also be used as an isolated procedure for induction, provided the cervical score is favorable [38].

Compared with oxytocin induction, recent trial studies have suggested that membrane stripping increased the rate of spontaneous vaginal delivery and shortened the induction to delivery interval [57].

Giving the potential risks of membrane rupture and associated maternal and neonatal infection, undertaking membrane stripping should be carefully weighed before performing the procedure in known GBS carriers [58, 59].

Prerequisite for membrane stripping: In order to use membrane stripping for induction or as a cervical ripening agent, there are criteria that need to be fulfilled. These are:

a. The fetal head must be well applied to the cervix.

b. The cervix should be dilated so as to allow the introduction of the examiner's finger [38].

Advantage and limitation of membrane stripping

- It has low cost than other pharmacological methods [60].
- It has an increased risk of vaginal bleeding and discomfort during vaginal examination compared with expectant management.

6.2.2 Balloon devices: Foley Catheter

Another non-pharmacological option for labor induction is the insertion of balloon catheter, which includes the introduction of a single or a double balloon catheter under sterile technique into the intracervical canal past the internal os. The bulb is then inflated with 30–60 cc of water, and it applies pressure on the internal os of the cervix to stretch the lower uterine segment and increase the release of local PG [32].

The catheter is left in place until either it falls out spontaneously or 24 hours have elapsed. Some practitioners apply a small degree of traction on the catheter by taping it to the inside of the leg [61].

Limitation of balloon device

- The insertion of balloon devices is contradicted in the presence of low-lying placenta
- Its use is relative contraindicated in the presence of antepartum hemorrhage, rupture of membranes, and evidence of lower tract genital infection [32].

6.2.3 Artificial rupture of membranes (AROM)

Amniotomy, also known as artificial rupture of membranes (AROM), is the intentional rupture of this amniotic sac by an obstetrical provider. This procedure is common during labor management and has been performed by obstetrical providers for quite a long time. The principal reasons for artificial rupture of membranes are to ripen the cervix, induce or augment the labor process, and assist in the placement of internal fetal monitoring devices to provide the direct assessment of fetal status [32, 62–64].

Rupture of the membranes causes cervical ripening and labor onset by different mechanisms, which include stretching of the cervix, separation of the membranes (liberation of prostaglandins), and reduction of amniotic fluid volume.

The effectiveness of ARM depends on the state of the cervix, station of the presenting part, and use of other methods, with shorter induction delivery interval when amniotomy is combined with oxytocin than used singly [38].

Advantages of amniotomy

- High success rate
- Chance to observe the amniotic fluid for blood or meconium

- Access to use fetal scalp electrode or intrauterine pressure catheter or for fetal scalp blood sampling

- Furthermore, other than causing cervical ripening and inducing labor, artificial rupture of membranes has other immediate benefits [38], such as lowering of the blood pressure in preeclampsia and relief of maternal distress in hydramnios.

Limitations

- Once the procedure is adopted, there is no scope of retreating from the decision of delivery.

- It cannot be employed in closed cervix. The cervix should be at least one finger dilated.

Contraindications

Use of ARM for labor induction and cervical ripening is contraindicated in the presence of the following conditions:

- Closed cervix

- Presenting part not engaged: if the presenting part is not engaged doing ARM may increase the risk of cord prolapse.

- Intrauterine fetal death

- Complete placenta previa

- Transverse lie: it increases the risk of cord prolapse

- Breech presentation prior to full dilation

- Maternal AIDS and active genital herpes infection: to reduce the risk of mother-to-child transmission

- It is also preferably avoided in chronic hydramnios, as there is risk of sudden massive liquor drainage and uterine decompression that may lead to early placental separation. In such a case, if necessary, controlled ARM should be done.

Risks and Complications of ARM

The most common complication of artificial rupture of membranes is prolapse of the umbilical cord. This invariably occurs if artificial rupture of membranes is performed before the head is engaged in the maternal pelvis [38]. Additional ARM have the following risks and complications:

- Uncontrolled escape of amniotic fluid and placental abruption

- Injury to the cervix or the presenting part

- Rupture of vasa praevia leading to fetal blood loss

- Amnionitis
- Accidental injury to the placenta, cervix or uterus, fetal parts, or vasa previa
- Liquor amni embolism (rare).

6.3 Combined Methods

Having a lack of most established single effective method for inducing labor in the obstetrics literatures, combined methods have been implemented to increase the success rate of induction [65, 66]. Combined method could be using either more than one medical methods or medical methods with mechanical methods. The most commonly used combined methods for induction are the use of oxytocin infusion that could be started either prior to or following prostaglandins or rupture of the membranes depending mainly upon the state of the cervix and head brim relation [38]. The advantages of the combined methods are:

1. More effective than any single procedure
2. Shortens the induction-delivery interval and thereby minimizes
    - The risk of infection and
    - The period of observation.

Conflict of interest

The authors declare no conflict of interest.

Acronyms and abbreviations

APGAR	appearance, pulse, grace, activity, reflex
ARM	artificial rupture of membranes
CEMOC	comprehensive emergency obstetric care
CS	cesarean section
FIOL	failed induction of labor
ICU	intensive care unit
IOL	induction of labor
IUFD	intrauterine fetal death
IUGR	intrauterine growth restriction
NICU	neonatal intensive care unit
PG	prostaglandin
PIH	pregnancy-induced hypertension
PPH	postpartum hemorrhage
PPROM	preterm premature rupture of the membranes
PROM	premature rupture of the membranes
SDG	sustainable development goal

Author details

Mulugeta W. Arage
Wodia University, Woldia, Ethiopia

*Address all correspondence to: mulewodaje@gmail.com

References

[1] Caughey AB, Sundaram V, Kaimal AJ, Cheng YW, Gienger A, Little SE, et al. Maternal and neonatal outcomes of elective induction of labor. Evidence Report/Technology Assessment. 2009; **176**:1

[2] Organization WH. WHO Recommendations for Induction of Labour. Geneva: World Health Organization; 2011

[3] Cunningham F, Leveno K, Bloom S, Spong CY, Dashe J. Williams Obstetrics. 24th ed. Mcgraw-Hill; 2014

[4] Sujata P, Chanania K, Hansa J, Chanania K. Comparative study between elective induction of labour and spontaneous labour. Advances in Bioresearch. 2017;**8**(2)

[5] Abdulkadir D, Geremew DW. Induction of labor prevalence and associated factors for its outcome at Wolliso St. Luke, Catholic Hospital, South West Shewa, Oromia. Internal Medicine. 2017;7:255

[6] Jacquemyn Y, Michiels I, Martens G. Elective induction of labour increases caesarean section rate in low risk multiparous women. Journal of Obstetrics and Gynaecology. 2012;**32**(3): 257-259

[7] Unicef. Levels & Trends in Child Mortality: Report 2010: Estimates Developed by the UN Inter-Agency Group for Child Mortality Estimation. United Nation Childrens Fund; 2017

[8] Vogel JP, Gülmezoglu AMM, Hofmeyr GJ, Temmerman M. Global perspectives on elective induction of labor. Clinical Obstetrics and Gynecology. 2014;**57**(2):331-342

[9] Abisowo O, Oyinyechi A, Olusegun F, Oyedokun O, Motunrayo A, Abimbola O. Feto-maternal outcome of induced versus spontaneous labour in a Nigerian tertiary maternity unit. Tropical Journal of Obstetrics and Gynaecology. 2017;**34**(1):21

[10] Alkema L, Chou D, Hogan D, Zhang S, Moller A-B, Gemmill A, et al. Global, regional, and national levels and trends in maternal mortality between 1990 and 2015, with scenario-based projections to 2030: A systematic analysis by the UN Maternal Mortality Estimation Inter-Agency Group. The Lancet. 2016;**387**(10017):462-474

[11] Saccone G, Berghella V. Induction of labor at full term in uncomplicated singleton gestations: A systematic review and metaanalysis of randomized controlled trials. American journal of Obstetrics and Gynecology. 2015;**213**(5): 629-636

[12] Girma W, Tseadu F, Wolde M. Outcome of induction and associated factors among term and post-term mothers managed at Jimma University specialized hospital: A two years' retrospective analysis. Ethiopian Journal of Health Sciences. 2016;**26**(2):123-132

[13] Zenzmaier C, Leitner H, Brezinka C, Oberaigner W, König-Bachmann M. Maternal and neonatal outcomes after induction of labor: A population-based study. Archives of Gynecology and Obstetrics. 2017;**295**(5):1175-1183

[14] Oyebode TA, Toma BO, Shambe IH, Kahansim ML, Embu HY, Daru PH, et al. Induction of labour at Jos University teaching, hospital, Jos, Nigeria: A four year review. International Journal of Research in Medical Sciences. 2017;**3**(8): 1942-1948

[15] Gill P, Lende MN, Van Hook JW. Induction of labor. StatPearls; 2022

[16] Obstetricians ACo, Gynecologists. ACOG committee opinion no. 560: Medically indicated late-preterm and early-term deliveries. Obstetrics and Gynecology. 2013;**121**(4):908-910

[17] Patabendige M, Jayawardane A. Foley catheter for cervical priming in induction of labour at University Obstetrics Unit, Colombo, Sri Lanka: A clinical audit with a patient satisfaction survey. BMC Research Notes. 2017; **10**(1):155

[18] González-Maestro M, Laurrieta-Saiz I, García-González C, López-Mirones M, Terán-Muñoz O, Alonso-Salcines A. Características de los partos inducidos en el Hospital Universitario Marqués de Valdecilla. Enfermeria Clinica. 2017; **2017**

[19] Tandu-Umba B, Tshibangu RL, Muela AM. Maternal and perinatal outcomes of induction of labor at term in the university clinics of Kinshasa, DR Congo. Open Journal of Obstetrics and Gynecology. 2013;**3**(01):154

[20] Coyne L. Dewhurst's textbook of obstetrics & gynaecology. The Obstetrician & Gynaecologist. 2008; **10**(1):66

[21] Batinelli L, Serafini A, Nante N, Petraglia F, Severi FM, Messina G. Induction of labour: Clinical predictive factors for success and failure. Journal of Obstetrics and Gynaecology: The Journal of the Institute of Obstetrics and Gynaecology. 2018;**38**(3):352-358

[22] Yosef T, Getachew D. Proportion and outcome of induction of labor among mothers who delivered in teaching hospital, Southwest Ethiopia. Frontiers in Public Health. 2021;**2021, 9**

[23] Bello FA, Akinyotu OO. Predictors of successful induction of labour at a tertiary obstetric service in Southwest Nigeria. Tropical Journal of Obstetrics and Gynaecology. 2016;**33**(2):143-148

[24] Tadesse T, Assefa N, Roba HS, Baye Y. Failed induction of labor and associated factors among women undergoing induction at University of Gondar Specialized Hospital, Northwest Ethiopia. BMC Pregnancy and Childbirth. 2022;**22**(1):175

[25] Khan NB, Ahmed I, Malik A, Sheikh L. Factors associated with failed induction of labour in a secondary care hospital. Journal of the Pakistan Medical Association: JPMA. 2012;**62**(1):6

[26] Frederiks F, Lee S, Dekker G. Risk factors for failed induction in nulliparous women. The Journal of Maternal-Fetal & Neonatal Medicine. 2012;**25**(12): 2479-2487

[27] Debele TZ, Cherkos EA, Badi MB, Anteneh KT, Demssie FW, Abdo AA, et al. Factors and outcomes associated with the induction of labor in referral hospitals of Amhara regional state, Ethiopia: A multicenter study. BMC Pregnancy and Childbirth. 2021;**21**(1): 1-8

[28] Cunningham FG, Leveno KJ, Bloom SL, Spong CY, Dashe JS. Williams Obstetrics. 24th ed. New York, Mcgraw-hill; 2014

[29] Rouse DJ, Weiner SJ, Bloom SL, Varner MW, Spong CY, Ramin SM, et al. Failed labor induction: Toward an objective diagnosis. Obstetrics and Gynecology. 2011;**117**(2 0 1):267

[30] Health FDRoEMo. Management Protocol on Selected Obstetric Topics. Federal Ministry of Health Addis Ababa; 2010

[31] Gabbe SG, Niebyl JR, Simpson JL, Landon MB, Galan HL, Jauniaux ER, et al. Obstetrics: Normal and Problem Pregnancies e-Book. Elsevier Health Sciences; 2016

[32] Dean Leduc M, Ottawa ON, Anne Biringer M, Toronto ON, Lily Lee M, Vancouver BC, et al. SOGC CLINICAL PRACTICE GUIDELINE.Induction of labour. Journal of Obstetrics and Gynaecology Canada. 2013;**9**(35): 840-857

[33] Tripathy P, Pati T, Baby P, Mohapatra SK. Prevalence and Predictors of Failed Induction

[34] Guerra G, Cecatti J, Souza J, Faundes A, Morais S, Gülmezoglu A, et al. Factors and outcomes associated with the induction of labour in Latin America. BJOG: An International Journal of Obstetrics & Gynaecology. 2009; **116**(13):1762-1772

[35] Knoche A, Selzer C, Smolley K. Methods of stimulating the onset of labor: An exploration of maternal satisfaction. Journal of Midwifery & Women's Health. 2008;**53**(4):381-387

[36] Wd A. Induction of labor. 2009

[37] Wormer KC, Bauer A, Williford AE. Bishop Score. StatPearls Publishing; 2021

[38] Konar H. DC Dutta's Textbook of Obstetrics. JP Medical Ltd; 2018

[39] Bishop EH. Pelvic Scoring for Elective Induction. 1964

[40] Brennand JE, Calder AA. Labor and normal delivery: Induction of labor. Current Opinion in Obstetrics & Gynecology. 1991;**3**(6):764-768

[41] Xenakis EM-J, Piper JM, Conway DL, Langer O. Induction of labor in the nineties: Conquering the unfavorable cervix. Obstetrics & Gynecology. 1997;**90**(2):235-239

[42] Xi M, Gerriets V. Prostaglandin E2 (Dinoprostone). 2019

[43] Mozurkewich EL, Chilimigras JL, Berman DR, Perni UC, Romero VC, King VJ, et al. Methods of induction of labour: A systematic review. BMC Pregnancy and Childbirth. 2011;**11**:84

[44] Calder A, Izm A. Review of Propess-a controlled release dinoprostone (prostaglandin E2) pessary. Journal of Obstetrics and Gynaecology: The Journal of the Institute of Obstetrics and Gynaecology. 1997;**17**(Suppl. 2):S53-S67

[45] Chatsis V, Frey N. Misoprostol for Cervical Ripening and Induction of Labour: A Review of Clinical Effectiveness, Cost-Effectiveness and Guidelines. 2019

[46] New U. Food and Drug Administration labeling on Cytotec (misoprostol) use and pregnancy. ACOG Committee Opinion No. 283. American College of Obstetricians and Gynecologists. Obstetrics and Gynecology. 2003;**101**:1049-1050

[47] Obstetricians ACo, Gynecologists. ACOG practice bulletin no. 107: Induction of labor. Obstetrics and Gynecology. 2009;**114**:386-397

[48] Hofmeyr G, Alfirevic Z, Matonhodze B, Brocklehurst P, Campbell E, Nikodem V. Titrated oral misoprostol solution for induction of labour: A multi-Centre, randomised trial. British Journal of Obstetrics and Gynaecology. 2001;**108**(9):952-959

[49] Wing DA, Rahall A, Jones MM, Goodwin TM, Paul RH. Misoprostol: An effective agent for cervical ripening and

labor induction. American journal of Obstetrics and Gynecology. 1995;**172**(6): 1811-1816

[50] Thomas J, Fairclough A, Kavanagh J, Kelly AJ. Vaginal prostaglandin (PGE2 and PGF2a) for induction of labour at term. Cochrane Database of Systematic Reviews. 2014;**6**

[51] Weeks A, Alfirevic Z, Faundes A, Hofmeyr G, Safar P, Wing D. Misoprostol for induction of labor with a live fetus. International Journal of Gynecology & Obstetrics. 2007;**99**:S194-S1S7

[52] Osilla EV, Sharma S. Oxytocin. StatPearls Publishing; 2021

[53] Blanks AM, Thornton S. The role of oxytocin in parturition. BJOG: An International Journal of Obstetrics & Gynaecology. 2003;**110**:46-51

[54] Kelly AJ, Tan BP. Intravenous oxytocin alone for cervical ripening and induction of labour. Cochrane Database of Systematic Reviews. 2001;**3**

[55] Hayes EJ, Weinstein L. Improving patient safety and uniformity of care by a standardized regimen for the use of oxytocin. American Journal of Obstetrics and Gynecology. 2008;**198**(6):622 e1-. e7

[56] O'Driscoll K, Foley M, MacDonald D. Active management of labor as an alternative to cesarean section for dystocia. Obstetrics & Gynecology. 1984;**63**(4):485-490

[57] Hapangama D, Neilson JP. Mifepristone for induction of labour. Cochrane Database of Systematic Reviews. 2009;**3**

[58] Boulvain M, Kelly A, Lohse C, Stan C, Irion O. Mechanical methods for induction of labour. The Cochrane Database of Systematic Reviews. 2001;(4):Cd001233

[59] Verani JR, McGee L, Schrag SJ. Prevention of perinatal group B streptococcal disease–revised guidelines from CDC, 2010. MMWR Recommendations and Reports : Morbidity and Mortality Weekly Report Recommendations and Reports. 2010;**59**(Rr-10):1-36

[60] Boulvain M, Stan CM, Irion O. Membrane sweeping for induction of labour. Cochrane Database of Systematic Reviews. 2005;**1**

[61] Leduc D, Biringer A, Lee L, Dy J, Corbett T, Duperron L, et al. Induction of labour. Journal of Obstetrics and Gynaecology Canada. 2013;**35**(9): 840-857

[62] Worthley M, Kelsberg G, Safranek S. Does amniotomy shorten spontaneous labor or improve outcomes? The Journal of Family Practice. 2018;**67**(12): 787-788

[63] ACOG Committee Opinion No. 766: Approaches to limit intervention during labor and birth. Obstetrics and Gynecology. 2019;**133**(2):e164-ee73

[64] Mahdy H, Glowacki C, Eruo FU. Amniotomy. StatPearls Publishing; 2021

[65] Faiz W, Skheel H, Abdulla K, Fawzi H, Alheshimi S. Combined versus single method for induction of labor. Iranian Journal of Public Health. 2020;**11**: 803

[66] Lovely NAA, Islam AT, Ali OI, Khatun R. Effect of combined medical and surgical induction of labour in term pregnancy at Rajshahi Medical College Hospital. TAJ: Journal of Teachers Association. 2018;**31**(2):17-20

Chapter 2

Vaginal Birth after Caesarean (VBAC)

Benjamin Joseph Nggada

Abstract

The rising rate of caesarean section has implications in the reproductive performance of a woman and increases the likelihood of complications during repeat operations, whether they are planned or performed on an emergency basis. A successful vaginal delivery after caesarean is associated with increased maternal satisfaction, reduced caesarean section rate, and appears to be cost effective. There is a need for careful selection of women that are willing to attempt vaginal birth after caesarean with a clear set of local protocols to increase overall success rate, reduce litigation and improve neonatal outcome. The benefits and risks of planned vaginal birth after caesarean and elective repeat caesarean section should be discussed in detail with the woman during antenatal care and reemphasized at admission to the labour ward. A decision to embark on VBAC should be free from coercion with full informed consent as the bedrock for such a decision. Facilities offering vaginal birth in women with prior caesarean delivery should be equipped with 24-hour standby emergency caesarean section capability. The intrapartum care should be carefully tailored to meet the woman's need with support from the health care team. Every obstetrics unit should debrief women after delivery irrespective of the outcome and should conduct regular audits to improve the care of women with previous caesarean sections.

Keywords: vaginal birth after caesarean (VBAC), elective repeat caesarean section (ERCS), trial of labour after caesarean (TOLAC), successful VBAC, uterine rupture

1. Introduction

Vaginal Birth After Caesarean (VBAC) is one of the most contentious topics in obstetrics, therefore physicians and health workers in maternal health must navigate the complexity of the pros and cons when advising and counselling prospective mothers that wish to consider the vaginal route of delivery after a caesarean [1]. The increased rates of caesarean section and the short- and long-term complications thereof have made VBAC a reasonable and cost-effective alternative to planned Elective Repeat Caesarean Section (ERCS) [2]. The single most common indication for Caesarean Delivery (CD) in several settings in both developing and developed countries is a previous caesarean section and VBAC has the potential to plateau or flatten the exponential trajectory of CD [3]. However, the contribution of VBAC is jeopardised by the current upsurge of Caesarean Delivery on Maternal Request

(CDMR), increased litigation climate and the cloud of caesarean sections that are generally classified as unnecessary by the World Health Organisation (WHO) [4–6]. The pendulum in the trend in VBAC and ERCS continues to swing back and forth with the debate concerning the acceptable ideal caesarean section rate persisting despite the recommendation by WHO. It is believed that the ideal caesarean section rate should be between 10 and 15% [7], however, in the recommendations by WHO to reduce unnecessary caesarean sections using nonclinical interventions, it was noted that these quoted rates are population based and that the panel conclusions were from temporally limited data in a European context [6]. The rising caesarean section rate has been deemed medically unnecessary and potentially harmful and it is predicted that nearly one third (29%) of all deliveries might be by caesarean section by 2030 [8]. In Latin America and the Caribbean, the proportion of caesarean section has outnumbered vaginal delivery and the projected rate by 2030 will likely to be 63, 54, 50 and 45% in Eastern Asia, Latin America and Caribbean, Western Asia and Australia and New Zealand respectively [8]. Therefore, it is pertinent to closely study the causes of high caesarean section rates with the aim of mitigating them, while encouraging VBAC as an alternative.

2. Evolution of VBAC

In 1916, Edwin B. Cragin in his classic publication on conservatism in obstetrics opined that once a caesarean delivery always a caesarean delivery which was later coined as the Dictum of Cragin. He argued that following surgical incision on the anterior abdominal wall and the uterine wall to deliver a fetus should rely on such method for future deliveries. In his article, he highlighted that the risk of uterine rupture is high in VBAC as the uterus is unable to withstand the shear stress of uterine contractions [9, 10]. The practice (of repeat caesarean delivery) was the standard of care until the late 1980s when its reputation was questioned by the National Institutes of Health in Bethesda, Maryland following an exponential surge in caesarean delivery rates and a review by the American Congress of clinical Obstetrics and Gynaecology which modified this recommendation and advocated that a woman can attempt vaginal delivery after one previous caesarean section [9, 11]. There has been remarkable progress in caesarean section techniques with Kerr's incision on the lower segment being the standard as opposed to the classical incision and caesarean section is now generally considered as a safe procedure with the risk of future uterine rupture considerably very low [12]. Evidence from systematic reviews and clinical guidelines suggest that planned VBAC is a safe and suitable method of delivery for most women after uncomplicated previous caesarean delivery [13–15].

3. Updated data

There is varied data across different settings concerning the rate of VBAC with several compounding factors. VBAC rates are generally reported to range from 49–87% [13]. In scrutiny of pregnancy outcomes following one previous caesarean section at Mafraq Hospital Abu Dhabi, Balachandran et al. [16] discovered that 76 percent were candidates for VBAC after careful patient selection and VBAC success rate was 83.47% with only 12.6% deemed to have failed VBAC. However, VBAC rates are said to be very low in low-income countries because of lack of facilities and manpower for adequate fetal monitoring [17]. In a recent Pretoria study VBAC rate is quoted be as low as 36% and lack of appropriate counselling on delivery options has been found to be a major culprit [18]. In a retrospective case study and online survey in Romania [19] VBAC rate was less than 1% which was attributable to lack of advocacy and promotion for VBAC, poorly trained health care workers and birth practices that favour repeat caesarean delivery, while average Europe VBAC rates are quoted to be between 20 and 50% [20].

4. Definition of terms

Vaginal Birth After Caesarean (VBAC): Vaginal delivery following one or more previous CD [21].

Planned VBAC: The Royal College of Obstetricians and Gynaecologists defined planned VBAC as an intended mode of delivery of any woman who previously had caesarean section (s) who opts to deliver vaginally instead of an Elective Repeat Caesarean Section (ERSC) [22].

Trial of Labour After Caesarean (TOLAC): This refers to the planned attempt to deliver vaginally following a previous caesarean birth, regardless of the outcome [23].

Successful VBAC: A vaginal delivery (spontaneous or assisted) following planned VBAC is termed as successful, whereas delivery by emergency caesarean section during the labour process is considered unsuccessful. Technically a vaginal delivery by a patient with previous caesarean section(s) even when not planned will be considered a successful VBAC [22, 23].

Elective Repeat Caesarean Section (ERCS): A planned caesarean delivery by a woman who had prior caesarean section(s).

Primary Caesarean Section: This is considered as the first delivery by caesarean section irrespective of the woman's parity [21–24].

Intervals

1. **Interpregnancy interval (IPI):** This is the time period between delivery of the last child and conception of the next pregnancy [25].

2. **Interdelivery interval:** The period of time from the last delivery to the onset of labour or a presumed expected date of delivery [26, 27].

Uterine rupture:

1. **Complete or symptomatic:** The complete disruption of the entire thickness of the uterine wall associated with extrusion of fetal parts and intraamniotic content in the peritoneal cavity [28, 29].

2. **Partial or uterine dehiscence:** This term is used when the uterine serosa is intact despite disruption of the uterine muscle [28, 29].

5. VBAC predictive factors

The success rate of planned VBAC has been quoted to be between 75 and 90% [22] and consensus from evidence-based guidelines and systematic reviews have endorsed

VBAC as a safe alternative for delivery for majority women with prior single lower segment CD, with a complication risk of less than 1% [14, 21–23]. Therefore, there is a need during prenatal care to carefully select women, counsel them appropriately and implement a VBAC checklist which will improve success and prevent complication and litigation [21, 22, 30]. Several factors have been found to positively predict successful VBAC and this should be carefully assessed during the entire prenatal care. Evidence based research has established the followings factors to impact positively on the success of VBAC:

5.1 Maternal will

Prospective parturient(s) who are well motivated to have VBAC after careful selection and counselling is associated with a positive outcome and higher chances of successful VBAC. This has been found to be critical in patients that undergo VBAC when compared to patients that are unwilling to try a vaginal delivery [21, 22, 31, 32].

5.2 Body Mass index < 30 kg/M2

VBAC success rate is inversely proportional to increasing BMI. VBAC rate decreases in obese women, however, appears unchanged in overweight women [33]. Weight fluctuation between pregnancy is correlated with decrease VBAC rates especially among women who had normal BMI in previous pregnancy [32].

5.3 Single previous lower segment caesarean delivery

The risk of uterine rupture associated with a single uncomplicated lower segment caesarean section is very rare. The likelihood of uterine rupture is approximately one in 200 (0.5%) women [21, 22]. Caution should be exercised in women who have had a complicated lower segment caesarean section despite insufficient data on extension or inverted T or a J incision. Recommended mode of delivery in these women should be decided on case-by-case basis with the woman fully aware of risk of uncertainty [21, 22, 33]. Previous classical uterine incision is associated with a higher risk (5% or greater) of uterine rupture; therefore, this incision type and previous uterine rupture are absolute contraindications to VBAC, and all such women should be offered elective repeat caesarean section [21, 34–36]. There is conflicting evidence on the likelihood of uterine rupture on women with two previous lower segment caesarean sections. Women with two previous uncomplicated lower segment caesarean deliveries have VBAC success rates of 62–75% which is like single lower segment caesarean sections especially among women with previous vaginal delivery or previous successful VBAC [32]. However, it is reasonable to err on the side of caution and offer such women elective repeat caesarean section due to the conflicting data.

5.4 Non recurrent indication for CS

Indication of the previous caesarean section can influence the outcome of VBAC. Non recurrent indications are associated with higher rates of successful VBAC. Sixty percent of women with cephalopelvic disproportion as the indication for previous caesarean delivery will achieve vaginal delivery, while 89% will achieve vaginal delivery for non-recurrent indications [32].

5.5 Previous successful vaginal birth before or after VBAC

Prior vaginal delivery is the strongest positive predictor of VBAC. VBAC Success rate in women with a prior vaginal delivery is documented to range between 75 and 85%, while a prior successful VBAC gives the maximum success rate of between 90 and 93% [21–23, 32, 37].

5.6 Adequate inter pregnancy or inter delivery interval

The hysterotomy exact mechanism of healing is still blur regeneration and fibrosis both entertained. According to Buhimschi et al. [38], the healing and visco-elastic behaviour of a surgically wounded myometrium depends on and varies with genetic and phenotypic properties. According to the CORONIS multicentered 3 year follow up randomised control trial, uterine rupture and uterine scar dehiscence following a single or double layer closure were similar in patient that had TOLAC [39]. Therefore, in a case to standardised caesarean section a single layer closure of the uterus is recommended [40]. The recommended optimal interval to guaranty uterine scar integrity and to reduce the risk of uterine is 6 and 18 months for interpregnancy and Interdelivery intervals respectively [27, 32]. However, a recent retrospective study recommended an Interdelivery interval of 24 months to attempt VBAC [26].

5.7 Singleton and cephalic presentation considered favourable for VBAC

There is high success rate in women attempting VBAC with a singleton fetus in cephalic presentation with estimated fetal weight of less than 4000 g, although there are studies to demonstrate that women undergoing TOLAC with one prior low transverse caesarean delivery with twin gestation have similar outcomes [21–23, 32]. TOLAC in twin gestation with no prior vaginal delivery is associated with very low successful VBAC rate following evidence from a recent cohort report [41]. However, the Royal College of Obstetricians and Gynaecologist threshold for estimated fetal weight is 3800 g [22].

5.8 Spontaneous onset of labor has better prognosis for VBAC

Spontaneous onset of labour in a woman who is planned for VBAC has been associated with higher success rates and less complications compared with artificial initiation or augmentation of uterine contractions. In a recent meta-analysis of observational studies oxytocin use was associated with higher rate of uterine rupture and recommended cautious monitoring of oxytocin use during TOLAC [42].

6. VBAC check list

A VBAC check list will enable obstetricians and physicians in women's health to carefully select patients, improve communications, and avoid litigation from possible acts of omission and lack of proper documentation (**Table 1**). Below is an example of Queensland Clinical Guideline for Vaginal birth after caesarean (VBAC) which was adopted by Royal College of Obstetricians and Gynaecologists (**Table 2**) [21, 22].

Queensland Clinical Guideline: Vaginal birth after caesarean (VBAC)

Appendix A: Example VBAC counselling checklist

An example checklist which can be used by clinicians when counselling women about birth after previous CS.

Contraindications for VBAC			**Tick when discussed**
Contraindications include: previous uterine rupture; history of classical caesarean section; contraindications to vaginal birth which apply regardless of history of caesarean (e.g. placenta praevia)			☐
If complex caesarean scar (e.g. inverted T or J), or history of multiple caesarean sections, seek expert advice			☐
Likelihood of VBAC		**VBAC rate**	
One previous caesarean section, no previous vaginal birth		72–75%*	☐
One previous caesarean section, at least one previous vaginal birth		85–90%*	☐
Induced labour, no previous vaginal birth, BMI greater than 30, previous caesarean for dystocia.		If all factors present, 40%	☐
***Maternal* risks of planned VBAC and ERCS**			
Risk	**Planned VBAC**	**ERCS**	
Uterine rupture*	0.5%	<0.02%	☐
**If uterine rupture occurs, 14–33% risk of hysterectomy and 6.2% risk of perinatal death*			
Serious complications in future pregnancies	Not applicable if VBAC	Increased likelihood of placenta praevia/morbidly adherent placenta	☐
Maternal mortality	0.004%	0.013%	☐
***Fetal* risks of VBAC and ERCS**			
Risk	**Planned VBAC**	**ERCS**	
Antepartum stillbirth beyond 39+0 weeks awaiting labour	0.1%	Not applicable if ERCS at 39 weeks	☐
Hypoxic ischaemic encephalopathy (HIE)	0.08%	<0.01%	☐
Perinatal mortality	0.13%	0.05%	☐
Intrapartum care recommendations			
Recommended continuous electronic fetal monitoring in labour			☐
One-on-one midwifery care			☐
Birth in suitable facility			☐
Written information leaflets provided: VBAC ☐ ERCS ☐ Other ☐			

Table 1.
Queensland Clinical Guideline Vaginal birth after caesarean (VBAC) which was adopted by Royal College of Obstetricians and Gynaecologists (RCOG) [21, 22].

7. VBAC predictive score

There are several predictive tools and models to improve the outcome of VBAC which are deployed into clinical practice. However, this will not substitute careful clinical selection and judgement. The Flamm and Geiger VBAC risk score is a simple

Appendix B: Example management plan checklist

Example plan which can be completed by clinician and woman to document plan for birth and potential circumstances which may arise.

Management plan in the event of...			
Preterm labour	☐ VBAC	☐ Emergency CS	
Spontaneous labour before ERCS date	☐ VBAC	☐ Emergency CS	☐ Depends on situation Provide details:
No spontaneous labour by 41 weeks	☐ Induction of labour Provide details below in induction of labour row		
	☐ ERCS Provide details:		
	☐ Expectant management Provide details:		
Details of induction of labour			
Use of oxytocin in labour			
ERCS booking details			
Additional comments			

Table 2.
Queensland Clinical Guideline Vaginal birth after caesarean (VBAC) which was adopted by Royal College of Obstetricians and Gynaecologists [21, 22].

Parameter(s)	History and clinical parameters	Scores
1. Maternal age	<40 years	2
	>40 years	0
2. Vaginal birth history	Before and after first caesarean	4
	After first caesarean	2
	Before first caesarean	1
	None	0
3. Indication for caesarean	Failure to progress	0
	Other reasons	1
4. Cervical effacement (%)	>75	2
	25–75	1
	<25	0
5. Cervical dilation at admission (cm)	>4	1
	<4	0

Table 3.
Flamm and Geiger model VBAC risk score [43].

and popular tool of prediction of successful VBAC which uses 5 parameters with scores allocated as shown in **Table 3** [43]. In an analysis of the predictiveness and positive correlation of the Flamm and Geiger scoring system in a prospective observational study, it was found that most women with scores of <3 at the time of admission had emergency caesarean section and successful VBAC accounted for only 16%, while score of >8 had a success VBAC rate of 100% and the authors concluded that the application of the Flamm and Geiger scoring gave a fair judgement of successful VBAC rates [43]. In a much larger recent study in a resource constraint setting, the Flamm and Geiger admission criteria had similar outcomes, however decision also included factors like estimated fetal weight, interpregnancy interval and gestational age [44]. The Maternal-Fetal Medicine Unit Network has a VBAC calculator which incorporated maternal height, weight, pre-pregnancy BMI and devoid of race which is ethnicity. The predictive score appears to be similar to the Flamm and Geiger model [45]. https://mfmunetwork.bsc.gwu.edu/PublicBSC/MFMU/VGBirthCalc/vagbirth.html

https://www.mdcalc.com/calc/3317/vbac-risk-score-successful-vaginal-delivery-flamm-model

8. VBAC versus ERSC

The risk versus benefit of VBAC and ERCS should be highlighted with full disclosure to any prospective mother who had a prior caesarean delivery. The decision for a mother to attempt either routes should be based on informed consent and be free from coercion.

The following are evidence-based benefits and risks for VBAC and ERCS (**Tables 4–7**):

Maternal [22, 23, 46]	**Fetal and neonatal** [21–23, 47]
• 75 chances of successful vaginal delivery	• Reduce risk of transient respiratory distress (2–3%)
• Shorter hospital stays	• Increase likelihood of breast feeding at birth and continued postpartum period
• Faster recovery	
• Reduce chances of ERCS in the future and increase likelihood of future vaginal birth	
• Increase maternal satisfaction	
• Reduce maternal mortality rate (4/100,000)	

Table 4.
Benefits of planned VBAC [21–23, 46].

Maternal [21–23, 48, 49]	**Fetal and neonatal** [21–23, 48, 49]
• Increase risk of emergency Caesarean delivery (25–28%) with more morbidity compared with ERCS	• Increase risk (0.1%) of antepartum still birth beyond 39 weeks while awaiting labour (similar rate in nulliparous women)
• 1 in 200 (0.5%) risk of uterine rupture (risk is higher with Augmentation and induction of labour)	• Increase risk (0.08%) of hypoxic ischaemic encephalopathy (HIE)
• Increase risk of anal sphincter injury in VBAC (5%) and increase to 39% in instrumental delivery. This is dependent on the birth weight	• Increase risk (0.04%) delivery related perinatal death

Table 5.
Risk of planned VBAC [21–23, 48, 49].

Maternal [21–23, 50, 51]	**Fetal and neonatal** [21–23, 50, 51]
• Extremely low risk (<0.02) of uterine rupture	• Reduce risk (0.01%) of HIE
• A known and planned delivery date and reduce likelihood of emergency caesarean section	• Lower rate (0.05%) of perinatal death
• In the short time- Reduces the risk of pelvic organ prolapse and urinary incontinence (this depends on the number of vaginal births)	
• Offers additional opportunity of sterilization if fertility is no longer desired. Counseling and consent should be performed at least 2 weeks before delivery because of high level of regrets compared with interval procedure	

Table 6.
Benefits of planned ERCS [21–23, 50, 51].

Maternal	Fetal and neonatal
• Reduce potential in future conception	• Decrease likelihood of breast feeding
• Long recovery	• Increase transient respiratory morbidity (4-5%)
• Increase likelihood of future caesarean delivery, placenta previa and placenta accreta spectrum	
• Increase risk of maternal death (13/100,000)	

Table 7.
Risk of planned ERCS [21–23, 50, 51].

9. Proposed guideline of MCH (Obstetrics division) for VBAC

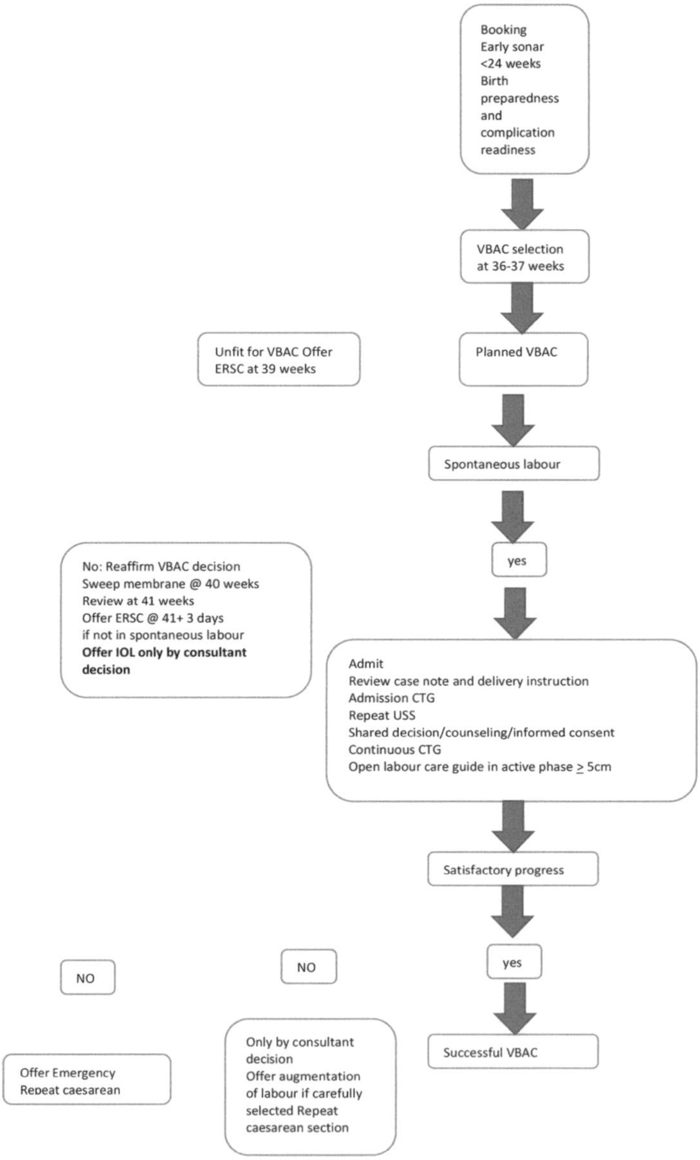

10. Intra partum monitoring of VBAC

Intrapartum monitoring for women undergoing TOLAC required a concise and structured plan to increase success rates, reduce morbidity and litigation from possible omission and lack of recognition of potential or actual uterine rupture. The maternity unit should be equipped with a standby 24-hour readiness for caesarean delivery with access to immediate neonatal care. The Obstetric team and the team leader preferably the unit consultant/the consultant on call should be notified immediately when a woman presents for a planned VBAC. All effort should be made to review all her case notes and the birth plan as documented during the antenatal care and allow the woman to reaffirm her decision to continue with the original plan or opt out for caesarean section [21–23]. It is appropriate to put in an intravenous canula and collect blood for a full blood count and blood group with the serum saved for access to immediate crossmatch if needed and oral intake should be restricted to clear fluid. The woman should be placed on continuous electronic fetal monitoring because an abnormal fetal rate is the most consistent finding in women who have uterine rupture [22, 51]. A one-to-one midwifery support and continuous care is associated with improve birth outcome and this should be the norm in all facilities that allow women to attempt vaginal delivery with prior caesarean. It is recommended to perform another vaginal examination once the woman is in active phase, open a labour care guide and repeat vaginal examinations every 4 hours. It is important to note that uterine rupture, which is the disruption of the uterine muscle, with or without the serosa [52] can occur at any stage of labour and they are no reliable clinical markers for early detection [22, 51, 52]. A prolonged and profound bradycardia correlates with more than 80% of uterine rupture. A classic triad of pain, vaginal bleeding and fetal heart abnormalities may only be present in about 10% of women and most likely a late sign. Nonspecific heart rate abnormalities might need to be interpreted in the context of the woman and other obstetrics conditions. However, the following nonspecific signs should be closely monitored. These are abdominal pain in-between contractions, acute onset of uterine scar tenderness, caseation of previously efficient uterine contractions, prolonged first or second stage of labour, haematuria, loss of station, easier palpation of fetal parts, shoulder tip or chest pain in absent of vaginal bleeding and evidence of maternal tachycardia and shock [22]. Where uterine rupture is suspected, the obstetrics team should aim at category 1 caesarean section. The third stage of labour should be managed based on local guideline for active management of the 3rd stage of labour. There are no contraindications to use of analgesia both systemic and regional in women during TOLAC [51].

11. VBAC in special clinical scenarios

Some clinical scenarios are a source of potential debate and management may vary according to local protocols, health workers experience, litigation climate and most importantly the women's preferences to mode of delivery.

11.1 Twin gestation

Uncomplicated twin gestation with the cephalic presentation in the leading twin has been found to have similar successful VBAC rates compared with singleton pregnancy [53–55]. However, caution should be taken for mother with twin gestation requesting for VBAC because of uncertainty regarding the safety of planned VBAC in these group of women. Ford et al. showed an increase (0.9%) scar rupture compared with the lower value in singleton with one previous lower segment scar [51, 55]. In a recent multicenter retrospective cohort study with a sample size of 160 women with twin A in vertex position with a single previous lower segment caesarean section, Peled et al. [56] stated that successful VBAC in selected twin was achieved in 86.3% while Levin et al. [41] reported a success VBAC rate of 31.3% in women with twins who attempted VBAC with no prior vaginal delivery.

11.2 Augmentation and induction of labour

Several studies [57, 58] have reported increased risk of uterine rupture in women who had either augmentation or induction of labour. However, there are inadequate and underpowered studies from randomised controlled trials concerning these clinical dilemmas. Therefore, when considering augmentation or induction of labour in patients with one prior lower segment caesarean section, the risks and benefits should be borne in mind by the clinician and discussed with the woman [51]. In an observational metanalysis of 14 studies [42] and a total of 48,457 women that underwent TOLAC, the rate of uterine rupture after induction was estimated to be about 2.2% which is which is a more than 4-fold increase in rate of uterine rupture when compared to an unstimulated uterus. Prostaglandins carry the greatest risk of rupture in comparison to mechanical methods and oxytocin augmentation. In a recent randomised trial to compare controlled release dinoprostone vaginal insert and foley's catheter for labour induction after one previous caesarean delivery, the induction delivery interval was shortened with dinoprostone, however, the rate of similar maternal satisfaction is similar [59]. The decision to stimulate the uterus either by artificial initiation or enhanced weak contraction in a patient undergoing TOLAC should be taken at the highest level of seniority, preferably by a specialist obstetrician.

11.3 Two or more previous CS

The outcome of planned VBAC in two or more prior caesarean sections is associated with low success rates and high rates of uterine rupture and greater catastrophic morbidity compared with women with one prior lower segment caesarean section [51]. The Royal College of Obstetricians and Gynaecologists cautiously states that VBAC can be considered in a pregnant woman at term with 2 previous uncomplicated lower segment caesarean sections after detailed informed consent by the consultant obstetrician but is contraindicated in a patient with 3 previous caesarean sections [22]. A case–controlled study that compared TOLAC and ERSC after 2 prior caesarean section found similar maternal and neonatal morbidity, however the uterine rupture rate was 1.16% compared with none in the ERSC group [60].

11.4 Preterm pregnancy

Preterm delivery in patients with prior caesarean section has been associated with lower success rates as reported in a multicenter trial retrospective study in preterm deliveries [61]. In patients with either fetal abnormalities or fetal demise in the mid trimester and prior caesarean section, options of hysterotomy, dilatation and curettage and medical induction of labour have not been randomised in any study [51].

Misoprostol has been reported to be successful in mid trimester termination of pregnancy for both women with and without previous caesarean section [62, 63]. A reasonable option is to use misoprostol and mifepristone, or a combination with intracervical balloon catheter can be carefully tailored to achieve vaginal delivery [51, 63].

11.5 Post date

There is evidence that the still birth rate at or after 39 weeks is higher (1.5–2-fold) in women with previous caesarean delivery compared to women with unscarred uterus. Data are not adequate to recommend delivery at this gestational age, more so that induction of labour is associated with reduced VBAC success rate and increased complications [22, 51]. If spontaneous labour has not occurred at 41 weeks, the RCOG recommends that the woman is reviewed by the senior obstetrician to reassess her options for membrane sweep, induction of labour or ERSC and provisional date for ERSC offered at 40 + 10 weeks. ACOG recognises that the likelihood of success VBAC may be less beyond 4o weeks but that should not be sole indication to preclude TOLAC [22, 23]. In a close analysis of gestational age and association with successful VBAC, Hackler et al. [64] found a bimodal distribution of high success rate between late preterm (34–36 weeks) and late term (41–42 weeks). The proportion of women that will experience spontaneous labour between 40 – 40 weeks +6 day is quoted to be more than 32% and 16% between 41 – 41 weeks +6 days [65]. Therefore, it would be reasonable to allow more than 40% of women to present in spontaneous labour if they desire to have a VBAC.

12. Contraindications to VBAC

Careful review of patient history, case notes, surgical notes, delivery plan and meticulous evaluation from prenatal care and at labour ward suit will help clinicians to tease out women that are not suitable for VBAC. Contraindications to VBAC are previous uterine rupture, classical caesarean section, and other contraindications to vaginal delivery like major degree placenta previa [21–23].

In a previous uterine rupture, there is a 5% or more recurrent rupture if vaginal delivery is attempted. There is insufficient evidence on the safety of VBAC in women who had a history of complicated scars like inverted T and J incisions and inadvertent uterine extension at primary incision, significant uterine surgery like myomectomy or any unification procedure, fetal macrosomia (estimated fetal weight > 3.8 kg) and breech presentation [21–23]. These complicated scars should be documented in the woman surgical notes and handcard and should be regarded as a contraindication to VBAC in future pregnancy. Maternal refusal should be considered an absolute contraindication to VBAC, and the prospective mother has the right to refuse VBAC during antenatal and intrapartum care. Epidural anaesthesia is not contraindicated in women with planned VBAC and should be offered to women on request where feasible [51].

13. Complications of VBAC

- The following complications for TOLAC and women who planned to have VBAC have been highlighted throughout the text and will be listed here for easy recall.

- Uterine rupture
- Major maternal morbidity (Hysterectomy, blood transfusion, genitourinary injuries)
- Maternal death
- Major perinatal morbidity (Fetal acidosis, HIE)
- Perinatal death

14. Conclusion

VBAC has clinical and public health importance with the overall aim of reducing caesarean section rate and its short- and long-term complications. There is a need to prevent unnecessary primary caesarean sections to curtail the alarmingly rising rates of caesarean sections in developing and developed countries. Women with a prior single lower segment caesarean section should be carefully selected during prenatal care and offered the option of planned VBAC. The use of check list, VBAC predictive score and scrutiny of surgical and clinical notes is a safe way to carefully select prospective mothers and improve VBAC success rates and eliminate complications related to VBAC. Every facility should implement regular audits to reflect on case management, improve patient selection and VBAC success rate.

Note

The author appreciates Dr. Tafadzwa Hazel Marufu for typesetting and assist in proof reading.

Author details

Benjamin Joseph Nggada
Department of Maternal and Child Health, University of Namibia, Windhoek, Namibia

*Address all correspondence to: bilyaminu@hotmail.com

References

[1] Handa M, Robertson A. Vaginal Birth After cesarean section: Ethical considerations for midwives. Canadian Journal of Midwifery Research and Practice. 2014;**13**(2):36-46 Available from: http://www.cjmrp.com/files/v13n2_commentary_vbac1.pdf

[2] Fobelets M, Beeckman K, Faron G, Daly D, Begley C, Putman K. Vaginal birth after caesarean versus elective repeat caesarean delivery after one previous caesarean section: A cost-effectiveness analysis in four European countries. BMC Pregnancy and Childbirth. 2018;**18**:92. DOI: 10.1186/s12884-018-1720-6

[3] Birara M, Gebrehiwot Y. Factors associated with success of vaginal birth after one caesarean section (VBAC) at three teaching hospitals in Addis Ababa, Ethiopia: A case control study. BMC Pregnancy and Childbirth. 2013;**13**:31. DOI: 10.1186/1471-2393-13-31

[4] Deng R, Tang X, Liu J, Gao Y, Zhong X. Cesarean delivery on maternal request and its influencing factors in Chongqing, China. BMC Pregnancy Childbirth. 2021;**21**:384. DOI: 10.1186/s12884-021-03866-7

[5] Yang YT, Mello MM, Subramanian SV, Studdert DM. Relationship between malpractice litigation pressure and rates of cesarean section and vaginal birth after cesarean section. Medical Care. 2009;**47**:234-242

[6] World Health Organization. WHO recommendations for non-clinical interventions to reduce unnecessary caesarean section. 2018. Available from: https://www.apps.who.int/iris/rest/bitstreams/1156517/retrieve

[7] World Health Organization. WHO statement on Caesarean section rates. 2015. Available from: https://www.apps.who.int/iris/rest/bitstreams/714841/retrieve

[8] World Health Organization. Caesarean section rates continue to rise, amid growing inequalities in access. 2021. Available from: https://www.who.int/news/item/16-06-2021-caesarean-section-rates-continue-to-rise-amid-growing-inequalities-in-access

[9] Cragin E. Conservatism in obstetrics. New York Medical Journal. 1916;**104**:1-3

[10] Sarah F. Conservatism in obstetrics. In: Cragin EB, editor. Embryo Project Encyclopedia (2017-04-11). 1916. ISSN: 1940-5030 Available from: http://www.embryo.asu.edu/handle/10776/11473

[11] Cunningham FG, Bangdiwala S, Brown SS, Dean TM, Frederiksen M, Rowland Hogue CJ, et al. National Institutes of Health Consensus Development Conference Statement: Vaginal Birth After Cesarean: New Insights. Obstetrics & Gynecology. 2010;**115**(6):1279-1295

[12] Bolla D, Schöning A, Drack G, Hornung R. Technical aspects of the caesarean section. Gynecological Surgery. 2010;**7**:127-132

[13] Guise JM, Eden K, Emeis C, Denman MA, Marshall N, Fu R, et al. Vaginal birth after cesarean: New Insights. Evidence Reports/Technology Assessments, No. 191. Rockville, Maryland, USA: Agency for Healthcare Research and Quality; 2010

[14] Dodd JM, Crowther CA, Huertas E, Guise JM, Horey D. Planned elective repeat caesarean section versus planned vaginal birth for women with a previous caesarean birth. Cochrane Database of

Systematic Reviews. 2004;(4): CD004224. DOI: 10.1002/14651858. CD004224.pub2

[15] Landon MB, Hauth JC, Leveno KJ, Spong CY, Leindecker S, Varner MW, et al. National institute of child health and human development maternal–fetal medicine units network. Maternal and perinatal outcomes associated with a trial of labor after prior cesarean delivery. The New England Journal of Medicine. 2004;**351**:2581-2589

[16] Balachandran L, Vaswani PR, Mogotlane R. Pregnancy outcome in women with previous one caesarean section. Journal of Clinical and Diagnostic Research. 2014;**8**(2):99-102. DOI: 10.7860/JCDR/2014/7774.4019

[17] Wanyonyi S, Muriithi FG. Vaginal birth after caesarean section in low resource settings: The clinical and ethical dilemma. Journal of Obstetrics and Gynaecology Canada. 2015;**37**(10): 922-926

[18] Masina T, Soma-Pillay P. Factors affecting VBAC success at a tertiary level hospital in Pretoria South Africa. Obstetrics and Gynaecology Forum. 2021;**31**(1):13-16

[19] Carauleanu A, Tanasa IA, Nemescu D, Haba R, Socolov D. Vaginal birth after Cesarean experience in Romania: A retrospective case-series study and online survey. Experimental and Therapeutic Medicine. 2021;**22**(2):894. DOI: 10.3892%2Fetm.2021.10326

[20] Lundgren I, Smith V, Nilsson C, Vehvilainen-Julkunen K, Nicoletti J, Devane D, et al. Clinician-centered interventions to increase vaginal birth after caesarean section (VBAC): A systematic review. BMC Pregnancy and Childbirth. 2015;**15**:16. DOI: 10.1186/ s12884-015-0441-3

[21] Queensland Clinical Guidelines. Vaginal birth after caesarean (VBAC). Guideline No. MN20.12-V5-R25. Queensland Health. 2020. Available from: http://www.health.qld.gov.au/qcg

[22] Royal College of Obstetricians and Gynaecologists. Birth after previous caesarean birth: Green-top guideline no. 45. [Internet] 2015. Available from: http://www.rcog.org.uk

[23] American College of Obstetricians and Gynecologists (ACOG). ACOG Practice Bulletin No. 205: Vaginal Birth After Cesarean Delivery. Obstetrics & Gynecology: 2019;**133**(2):e110-e127 DOI: 10.1097/AOG.0000000000003078

[24] Di Giovanni P, Garzarella T, Di Martino G, Schioppa FS, Romano F, Staniscia T. Trend in primary caesarean delivery: A five-year experience in Abruzzo, Italy. BMC Health Services Research. 2018;**18**:514. DOI: 10.1186/ s12913-018-3332-2

[25] Ndaninginan LL, Mlay P, Gaffur R, Nggada BJ, Mahande MJ. Effect of interpregnancy Interval on adverse maternal and perinatal outcomes at Katutura regional referral hospital in Namibia: A retrospective cohort study, 2005-2015. Acta Scientific Women's Health. 2020;**2**(12):2-9. DOI: 10.31080/ ASWH.2020.02.0161

[26] Rao J, Fan D, Ma H, Lin D, Zhang H, Zhou Z, et al. Is there an optimal inter-delivery interval in women who underwent trial of labor after cesarean delivery (TOLAC)? Reproductive Health. 2022;**19**:14. DOI: 10.1186/ s12978-021-01319-0

[27] American College of Obstetricians and Gynecologists. Society for maternal-fetal medicine. Obstetric care consensus No. 8 (Reaffirmed 2021): Interpregnancy care. Obstetrics and Gynecology. 2019;

133(1):e51-e72. DOI: 10.1097/AOG.0000000000003025

[28] Manoharan M, Wuntakal R, Erskine K. Uterine rupture: A revisit. The Obstetrician & Gynaecologist. 2010; **12**:223-230

[29] Abrar S, Abrar T, Sayyed E, Naqvi SA. Ruptured uterus: frequency, risk factors and feto-maternal outcome: Current scenario in a low-resource setup. PLoS One. 2022;**17**(4):e0266062. DOI: 10.1371/journal.pone.0266062

[30] Wu Y, Kataria Y, Wang Z, Ming WK, Ellervik C. Factors associated with successful vaginal birth after a cesarean section: a systematic review and meta-analysis. BMC Pregnancy and Childbirth. 2019;**19**(1):360. DOI: 10.1186%2Fs12884-019-2517-y

[31] David D, Homer CS, Clark D, Sabera T, Foureur M. Choosing vaginal birth after caesarean: motivating factors. Midwifery. 2020;**88**:102766. DOI: 10.1016/j.midw.2020.102766

[32] Trojano G, Damiani GR, Olivieri C, Villa M, Malvasi A, Alfonso R, et al. VBAC: Antenatal predictors of success. Acta Bio-Medica. 2019;**90**(3):300-309. DOI: 10.23750%2Fabm.v90i3.7623

[33] Karavani G, Chill HH, Reuveni-Salzman A, Guedalia J, Menahem-Zidon OB, Cohen N, et al. Risk factors for uterine incision extension during cesarean delivery. The Journal of Maternal-Fetal & Neonatal Medicine. 2022;**35**(11):2156-2161. DOI: 10.1080/14767058.2020.1783230

[34] Landon MB, Hauth JC, Leveno KJ, Spong CY, Leindecker S, Varner MW, et al. Maternal and perinatal outcomes associated with a trial of labor after prior cesarean delivery. New England Journal of Medicine. 2004;**351**(25):2581-2589

[35] Shipp TD, Zelop CM, Repke JT, Cohen A, Caughey AB, Lieberman E. Intrapartum uterine rupture and dehiscence in patients with prior lower uterine segment vertical and transverse incisions. Obstetrics and Gynecology. 1999;**94**(5 Pt 1):735-740

[36] Naef RW 3rd, Ray MA, Chauhan SP, Roach H, Blake PG, Martin JN Jr. Trial of labor after cesarean delivery with a lower-segment, vertical uterine incision: is it safe? American Journal of Obstetrics and Gynecology. 1995;**172**(6):1666-1673 discussion 73-4

[37] Sahin S, Ozkaya E, Eroglu M, Sanverdi I, Celik Z, Cakiroglu A. Predictors of successful vaginal birth after a caesarean in women with a previous single caesarean delivery. European Review for Medical and Pharmacological Sciences. 2022;**26**(5): 1594-1600. DOI: 10.26355/eurrev_202203_28226

[38] Buhimschi CS, Zhao G, Sora N, Madri JA, Buhimschi I. Myometrial wound healing post-cesarean delivery in the MRL/MpJ mouse model of uterine scarring. The American Journal of Pathology. 2010;**177**(1):197-207. DOI: 10.2353/ajpath.2010.091209

[39] CORONIS Collaborative Group, Abalos E, Addo V, Brockle-hurst P, El Sheikh M, Farrell B, et al. Caesarean section surgical techniques: 3 year follow-up of the CORONIS fractional, factorial, unmasked, randomised controlled trial. Lancet. 2016;**388**:62-72

[40] Dahlke JD, Mendez-Figueroa H, Maggio L, Sperling JD, Chauhan SP, Rouse DJ. Standardizing cesarean delivery technique. Obstetrics and Gynecology. 2020;**136**:972-980. DOI: 10.1097/AOG.0000000000004120

[41] Levin G, Yagel S, Schwartz A, Many A, Rosenbloom JI, Yinon Y, et al.

Trial of labor after cesarean in twin gestation with no prior vaginal delivery – evidence from largest cohort reported. International Journal of Gynecology & Obstetrics. 2022;**159**:229-236. DOI: 10.1002/ijgo.14090

[42] Zhang H, Liu H, Luo S, Weirong GU. Oxytocin use in trial of labor after cesarean and its relationship with risk of uterine rupture in women with one previous cesarean section: A meta-analysis of observational studies. BMC Pregnancy and Childbirth. 2021;**21**:11. DOI: 10.1186/s12884-020-03440-7

[43] Sahu R, Chaudhary N, Sharma A. Prediction of successful vaginal birth after caesarean section based on Flamm and Geiger scoring system a prospective observational study. International Journal of Reproduction, Contraception, Obstetrics and Gynecology. 2018;**7**: 3998-4002

[44] Mishra P, Mukherjee S, Gupta A, Aparajeeta. Analytical study on trial of scar using Flamm and Geiger admission scoring system for VBAC. International Journal of Contemporary Medical Research. 2020;**7**(1):A1-A4

[45] Grobman WA, Sandoval G, Rice MM, Bailit JL, Chauhan SP, Costantine MM, et al. Prediction of vaginal birth after cesarean delivery in term gestations: A calculator without race and ethnicity. American Journal of Obstetrics and Gynecology. 2021;**225**(664):e1-e7. DOI: 10.1016/j.ajog.2021.05.021

[46] Spong CY. To VBAC or not to VBAC. PLoS Medicine. 2012;**9**(3): e1001191. DOI: 10.1371/journal.pmed.1001191

[47] Regan J, Thompson A, DeFranco E. The influence of mode of delivery on breastfeeding initiation in women with a prior cesarean delivery: A population-based study. Breastfeeding Medicine. 2013;**8**:181-186

[48] Manresa M, Pereda A, Bataller E, Terre-Rull C, Ismail KM, Webb SS. Incidence of perineal pain and dyspareunia following spontaneous vaginal birth: A systematic review and meta-analysis. International Urogynecology Journal. 2019;**30**(6): 853-68.32

[49] Elvander C, Ahlberg M, Edqvist M, Stephansson O. Severe perineal trauma among women undergoing vaginal birth after cesarean delivery: A population-based cohort study. Birth. 2019;**46**(2): 379-386

[50] Fitzpatrick KE, Quigley MA, Kurinczuk JJ. Planned mode of birth after previous cesarean section: A structured review of the evidence on the associated outcomes for women and their children in high-income setting. Frontiers in Medicine. 2022;**9**:920647. DOI: 10.3389/fmed.2022.920647

[51] Royal Australian and New Zealand College of Obstetricians and Gynaecologist (RANZCOG). Birth after previous caesarean section. (C-Obs 38) Version 3.1 March 2019. Available from: https://www.ranzcog.edu.au/wp-content/uploads/2022/05/Birth-after-previous-caesarean-section.pdf

[52] Figueirolo-Filho EA, Gomez JM, Farine D. Risk factors associated with uterine rupture and dehiscence: a cross-sectional Canadian study. Revista Brasileira de Ginecologia e Obstetrícia. 2021;**43**(11):820-825

[53] Aaronson D, Harlev A, Sheiner E, Levy A. Trial of labor after cesarean section in twin pregnancies: maternal and neonatal safety. The Journal of Maternal-Fetal & Neonatal Medicine. 2010;**23**:550-554

[54] Cahill A, Stamilio DM, Paré E, Peipert JP, Stevens EJ, Nelson DB, et al. Vaginal birth after cesarean (VBAC) attempt in twin pregnancies: is it safe? American Journal of Obstetrics and Gynecology. 2005;**193**:1050-1055

[55] Ford AA, Bateman BT, Simpson LL. Vaginal birth after cesarean delivery in twin gestations: A large, nationwide sample of deliveries. American Journal of Obstetrics and Gynecology. 2006;**195**: 1138-1142

[56] Peled T, Sela HY, Joseph J, Martinotti T, Grisaru-Granovsky S, Rottenstreich M. Factors associated with failed trial of labor after cesarean, among women with twin gestation—A multicenter retrospective cohort study. Journal of Clinical Medicine. 2022;**11**: 4256. DOI: 10.3390/jcm11154256

[57] Kehl S, Weiss C, Rath W. Balloon catheters for induction of labor at term after previous cesarean section: A systematic review. European Journal of Obstetrics and Gynecology and Reproductive Biololgy. 2016;**204**:44-50

[58] Fitzpatrick KE, Kurinczuk JJ, Alfirevic Z, Spark P, Brocklehurst P, Knight M. Uterine rupture by intended mode of delivery in the UK: A national case-control study. PLoS Medicine. 2012; **9**(3):e1001184

[59] Sulaiman S, Sivaranjani S, Razali N, Lim BK, Hamadan M, Tan PC. Foley catheter compared with controlled release dinoprostone vaginal insert for labor induction after one previous cesarean delivery: A randomized trial. International Journal of Gynaecology and Obstetrics. 2022 July 23. DOI: 10.1002/ijgo.14364

[60] Horgan R, Hossain S, Fulginiti A, Patras A, Massaro R, Abuhamad AZ, et al. Trial of labor after two cesarean sections: A retrospective case–control study. The Journal of Obstetrics and Gynaecology Research. 2022;**48**(10): 2528-2533. DOI: 10.1111/jog.15351

[61] Rotem R, Hirsch A, Barg M, Mor P, Michaelson-Cohen R, Rottensteich M. Trial of labor following cesarean in preterm deliveries: Success rates and maternal and neonatal outcomes: A multicenter retrospective study. Archives of Gynecology and Obstetrics. 2022. DOI: 10.1007/s00404-022-06746-3

[62] Goyal V. Uterine rupture in second-trimester misoprostol-induced abortion after cesarean delivery: A systematic review. Obstetrics and Gynecology. 2009;**113**(5):1117-1123

[63] Kücükgöz Gülec U, Urunsak IF, Eser E, Guzel AB, Ozgunen FT, Evruke IC, et al. Misoprostol for midtrimester termination of pregnancy in women with 1 or more prior cesarean deliveries. International Journal of Gynaecology and Obstetrics. 2013; **120**(1):85-87. DOI: 10.1016/j.ijgo.2012.08.013

[64] Hackler F, Serra A, Twedt R, Cheng Y, Caughey A. Gestational age and association with successful vaginal birth after caesarean. American Journal of Obstetrics & Gynecology. 2017; **216**(1):S94. DOI: 10.1016/j.ajog.2016.11.041

[65] National Institute for Health and Care Excellence (NICE). Inducing Labour. 2021. Available from: https://www.nice.org.uk/guidance/ng207

Section 2

Cesarean Section and Hypertensive Disorders, Diabetes and Co-Existing Diseases in Pregnancy

Chapter 3

Caesarean Section on Maternal Request

Neha Sethi, Rajeev Kumar Rajaratnam and Nadiah Abdullah

Abstract

Caesarean section on maternal request (CSMR) is performed in the absence of a standard medical/obstetrical indication in order to avoid vaginal delivery. Globally, there has been an upsurge in CS delivery, which necessitates the urgency to address maternal and foetal health implications, and long-term repercussions. Conceptually, the chapter aims to explore the determinants of increased CSMR, highlight its potential risks and benefits, and discuss the ethical, medico-legal concerns. Findings indicate that medical, psychological, psychosocial, economical, social and cultural determinants might serve as some of the potential influencing factors owing to this serious healthcare concern. Although CSMR has been linked to certain beneficial outcomes (e.g. reduced urinary incontinence and pelvic organ prolapse, reduced rate of PTSD and depression, and lesser intrapartum complications), it still imposes serious maternal (e.g. post-partum haemorrhage and infection, visceral damage, placenta accrete, placental abruption and complications in future pregnancy) and foetal adverse outcomes (stillbirth, asphyxia, respiratory distress and other pulmonary infections). Hence, future approaches and interventions should be directed towards mitigating clinically unrequired CS procedures due to medical malpractices, lack of awareness in women and the underlying determinants of elective CS.

Keywords: caesarean section, maternal request, benefits and risks, prevalence of CSMR

1. Introduction

Caesarean delivery is 'the birth of a foetus through incisions in the abdominal wall (laparotomy) and the uterine wall (hysterotomy)' [1]. Historically, caesarean delivery has been linked to a high rate of complications, often resulting in maternal death. However, caesarean sections are globally practiced in the advanced era of medicine to facilitate improved pregnancy outcomes [2, 3]. A caesarean section (CS or C-section) can be classed as either elective or emergency depending on its urgency and/or timing. A planned or elective caesarean section is performed before the onset of labour. Contrarily, an emergency C-section is a procedure performed before or during labour out of concern for the mother or the foetus [4].

In the absence of maternal or foetal indications for caesarean birth, vaginal delivery is safe and appropriate and should be advised, according to the American College of Obstetricians and Gynecologists' committee [5]. In addition, performing C-section in the absence of any medical indication is against the norms and guidelines of the World Health Organization (WHO). However, reports from the Global Network for Women's and Children's Health Research indicate an alarming increase in caesarean delivery rates, which is consistent with the global trend. One potential driver of the escalating rates is caesarean birth by maternal request [6].

Caesarean section on maternal request (CSMR) is defined as 'a procedure performed in the absence of a standard medical or obstetrical indication in order to avoid vaginal delivery' [7]. In the recent years, the number of caesarean deliveries has increased tremendously worldwide. A high caesarean section rate has become a pressing issue, which raises the concern on its implications to maternal health as well as long-term consequences. The growing trend in C-section rates has been attributed to changes in maternal characteristics and professional practice approaches, as well as to rising malpractice pressure and economic, organizational, social and cultural variables. Inequities in the use of surgery, both between and within nations, as well as the expenditures that unnecessary caesarean sections impose on financially strapped health systems, are additional issues and debates surrounding C-section [8]. Planning a favourable delivery route requires balancing the risks and advantages of any medical procedure, including CSMR and planned vaginal deliveries [9]. More importantly, it demands higher awareness among women regarding the risks and advantages of planned and unplanned C-sections using evidence-based information and updated recommendation from the National Institute for Health and Clinical Excellence (NICE) [10].

Therefore, this chapter aims to review the current stature of scientific literature in order to (i) explore and link the determinants of increased CSMR; (ii) highlight the potential risks and benefits of elective CS procedure; (iii) and discuss the ethical, medico-legal concerns surrounding this controversial health issue.

1.1 Prevalence of caesarean sections

According to the World Health Organization (WHO) data, the recommended CS delivery rate ranges between 10% and 15%, while rates exceeding 15% are considered medically unnecessary [5]. In recent decades, the use of C-sections has risen dramatically worldwide, especially in middle- and high-income countries, despite scarce evidence on significant maternal and perinatal benefits and the possible link between increasing CS rates and worsening health outcomes [8].

Globally, C-sections have been rising rapidly since the early 1990s. Approximately 21% of the entire world's births have been ceased by CS, ranging from 6% in low- and middle-income countries (LMICs) to 27% in the developed nations. Regionally, an increased rate is observed in Eastern Asia (35%), Central America (38%), North America and Oceania (32%). According to recently estimated projections, the cumulative rates may escalate further to 50% by 2030, accounting for a global CS prevalence of 29% [11].

According to a 2010 WHO survey, 27.3% of deliveries in Asian regions were caesarean sections, with these statistics being much higher in China since they have adopted the two-child policy [12]. These figures were surprisingly much higher than the advised rate of 10–15% by WHO. In fact, in the developing nations, private facilities perform C-sections on maternal requests twice more frequently than the public hospitals [13]. In Thailand, nearly 53% of obstetricians would consider C-section on maternal request [14]. Similarly, in a province in China, CSMR accounted for 8.42%

of CS delivery out of 36.01% of caesarean cases [15]. The overall caesarean section rate in Malaysia ranged from 18.8% to 31.5%, and the prevalence was unexpectedly much higher among low-risk women [16]. The following data show an upsurge in the number of C-sections performed globally and necessitates a review of current regulations and policies in clinical practice.

The prevalence of CSMR varies widely across different nations, ranging between 0.2% and 42% of all deliveries, although most studies reported a prevalence of <5%. The lack of information on birth certificates and discharge sheets limits the data availability since it fails to address CS on maternal request, while the study year and diverse characteristics of the study population affect the prevalence of CSMR [9].

1.2 Economic burden

The financial incentives linked to CS delivery are crucial factors to consider from a healthcare professional's perspective. In comparison with vaginal birth, CS delivery results in increased net profitability for healthcare providers [17]. A caesarean surgery or a difficult vaginal delivery can cost between US$50 and US$100, while a regular delivery at a hospital in underdeveloped regions of Africa and Latin America costs between US$10 and US$35.

According to the World Health Report 2010, 6 million non-medically indicated CS procedures were carried out in 2008, costing approximately $2.32 billion in the United States [18]. The increment in salary of healthcare providers might be one of the leading contributors to unnecessary CS births [19]. Non-medically indicated C-sections place a disproportionately higher financial burden on women and lead to adverse health implications. Medical costs are typically higher if CS procedures are performed at private healthcare facilities. In addition, CS necessitates a lengthier hospital stay, which increases healthcare expenditure and results in financial deprivation [17, 19].

1.3 Indications and recommendations

CS can be a significantly life-saving intervention for medically indicated cases [19]. In ideal circumstances, C-sections are performed when vaginal delivery (VD) is contradicted to protect the newborn and the mother from a potentially adverse event [11].

Medically adopted classifications for performing CS deliveries are 'based on primary clinical indications', 'the degree of urgency or absolute need for caesarean delivery' and 'Robson classification'. The Robson classification also known as the 'Ten Group Classification System (TGCS)' has been endorsed by the WHO as a 'global standard' tool for CS evaluation. It classifies CS into 10 mutually exclusive and exhaustive groups based on the category of the pregnancy, the previous obstetric record of the woman, the course of labour and delivery, and the gestational age of the pregnancy [20].

Caesarean sections are widely performed for various maternal or foetal indications. Obstructed labour (including a severely malformed pelvis and a failed attempt at labour), extensive antepartum haemorrhage, grade 3 or 4 placenta praevia, malpresentation (including transverse, oblique and brow) and uterine rupture are all absolute maternal indicators. Non-absolute indications include maternal request, 'precious' pregnancy and psychosocial signs such as failure to progress in labour (including prolonged labour), failed induction, previous caesarean delivery, genitourinary fistula or third-degree tear repair, antepartum haemorrhage, maternal medical diseases, severe preeclampsia or eclampsia, foetal compromise (including foetal distress, cord compression and severe intrauterine growth retardation) and breech presentation [3].

A recent study in China reported maternal request (23.38 %), foetal distress (22.73 %) and pregnancy complications (9.96 %) as the leading indications for CS [15].

The frequency of unnecessary caesarean births has considerably decreased due to foetal cardiac monitoring and blood collection procedures. In the absence of the aforementioned indications, a VD is considered safe, and it improves the mother's recuperative process as well as her caring ability and bonding with newborn. However, not all women prefer the conventional VD over a planned CS, possibly owing to social, cultural and psychological factors. Necessary information should be provided to women while choosing the most suitable and safest mode of delivery. Women who request for CS should be evaluated and given the appropriate counselling. It is prudent to consider the motivation behind her request since it directs the obstetrician to explore, counsel and prepare her for the desired mode of delivery. This is crucial as an operative abdominal delivery carries significant morbidities such as post-partum haemorrhage, anaesthetic complications, surgical site infections and thromboembolic events [21]. Owing to these issues, the obstetrician should look into specific risk factors such as age, parity, body mass index and past obstetric history [11]. A woman's reproductive plans and personal values should also be taken into consideration before opting for elective CS and/or CSMR.

Women who opt for CSMR should be delivered no earlier than 39 weeks of gestation unless there are other clinical indications. It is crucial for women to be well informed about the risks of placenta praevia, placenta accreta spectrum, intrauterine mortality and caesarean hysterectomy in subsequent pregnancies [4]. Therefore, it is essential to provide these women with adequate knowledge before they can make significant decisions and exercise their autonomy competently as patients. Instead of declining the CS request, the obstetrician should use sound judgement to cater to the patient's needs and maximize an improved health outcome.

2. Determinants of CS on maternal request

Globally, the number of caesarean deliveries has significantly increased in recent years. This situation demands an urgency to address the high CS rate since it may lead to maternal health implications and long-term repercussions. Medical, psychological and psychosocial, economical, social and cultural determinants might serve as some of the potential influencing factors owing to this serious healthcare concern.

Multiple factors account for women requesting a caesarean delivery. The perception of the community that a CS is an almost low-risk alternative to VD may very well contribute to the rising number of cases in recent years [22]. The most prevalent causes for CSMR are psychological. Tocophobia or 'fear of childbirth' is one of the major reasons contributing to CSMR. The estimated prevalence of severe tocophobia is 14%, which appears to have increased recently [23]. Primary tocophobia affects nullipara, while secondary tocophobia affects women with previous obstetric history [24].

Tocophobic women frequently perceive childbirth as a dread of labour pain, pelvic floor damage resulting in incontinence of the urine or foeces, fear of requiring an emergency surgical delivery, dreading child loss and facing a fear of being left alone while in labour [25]. Therefore, the most significant risk factors for secondary tocophobia are prior unpleasant overall birth experience, combined anxiety and depression, and poor social support [26]. Due to the unpredictable nature of labour and the vaginal birth process, women who have faced previous difficulties that resulted in emergency caesarean sections or instrumental deliveries may request a caesarean section [25].

Whereas some women choose CSMR to have a planned and organized delivery [25], career-oriented women are more likely to prefer elective CS since it is more convenient to have a scheduled birth. A multicentre study conducted in Brazil discovered that women with higher education levels and income are more likely to give birth via caesarean section [27]. In addition, some cultures' astrological beliefs may also impact the decision to undergo CSMR since they believe there is a lucky day for childbirth [28]. Women with advanced maternal age, prior miscarriages, infertility and assisted reproductive technology have demonstrated higher rates of CSMR [22, 29]. These women consider their first pregnancy to be 'precious' and therefore decide to have an elective C-section because they believe it will be safer for their child [30].

According to a systematically analysed review, there may be several social and individual factors that have contributed to the rise in C-section deliveries on maternal requests, for instance, the fear of labour pain and the perception of inequity and inadequate treatment [31]. Similarly, women who had previously undergone a C-section contributed to the highest CS delivery rate. Additionally, cultural considerations such as religious acceptance, societal views towards the procedures, prior experiences and encounters with medical experts also influence women to request an elective CS for non-medical reasons [32]. The choice of delivery is significantly influenced by the partners as well [33]. A study in China [34] highlighted five key psychosocial elements that influenced the choice of delivery method by women, and included level of education, financial situation, parity, anxiety, and confidence of lying-in (i.e. pre-/postpartum confinement). Other factors contributing to the rise in C-section deliveries include increased socio-economic status and diversity in the cultural and societal contexts. Women from higher socio-economic background delay childbearing until their late 30s to achieve higher education, build a career and establish financial security, which leads them to elective CS delivery. In addition, CS rates have been considerably higher among urban populations and private healthcare settings [5, 20].

3. Potential risks and benefits of elective CS

Over the last 10 years, CS rates in developed nations have increased considerably, leading to controversial debates regarding the benefits of planned procedures on maternal and neonatal health outcomes [3]. Evidence shows that CS procedures globally avert 2.9 million neonatal deaths and around 187,000 maternal deaths [11]. Although CS leads to a significant mortality reduction, nevertheless, non-medically indicated CS might increase the short- and long-term health hazards for both mother and child [8]. Post-partum haemorrhage and infection, visceral damage, placenta accrete and placental abruption are among the short-term risks, whereas obesity and asthma are long-term risks [20, 35]. Additionally, mothers with CS have greater rates of miscarriage, ectopic pregnancy and stillbirth in subsequent pregnancies. Uterine rupture, placental accrete and placental abruption are also more prevalent among mothers with a previous history of CS [11].

Data suggest that CS increases the baby's risk of developing asphyxia, respiratory distress and other pulmonary infections. Maternal mortality is higher with CS than VD in some settings, most likely due to the adoption of non-medically elective CS [5, 19]. Increased illness, injury, and short- and long-term disability have been often linked to CS. In some circumstances, an emergency hysterectomy may seem potentially necessary to manage severe post-partum haemorrhage. CS cases may result in chronic pain, delay in the initiation of breastfeeding and criticality in future pregnancies [36]. Past studies reported that CS presents with an increased risk of childhood illnesses by 5% and imposes higher risk to maternal health [5].

Non-medically indicated and/or CS on maternal request should not be promoted since it is a major surgery and involves significant risk compared with the conventional VD [19]. Multiple risk factors should be assessed before adopting the CS procedure to ensure better health of the mother and the baby. Maternal age, weight, parity, extended labour, HIV-positive status, previous CS, dystocia, breech presentation, placenta praevia and potential foetal complications are some significant risk factors to consider. Therefore, it is important to control these risk factors at individual level and then opt for elective CS [19].

Although CSMR has several risks, it has some notable benefits as well that should be highlighted. One of the essential goals of C-sections is to ensure improved maternal and neonatal outcomes [19]. Here are some of the benefits associated with a planned caesarean section.

3.1 Anxiety and depression

Stress and anxiety can adversely affect maternal well-being and their ability to care for the newborn. PTSD has been recognised as a possible consequence of childbirth with a prevalence between 2% and 7%, while post-partum depression has been found to be around 10% [24]. Women with severe tocophobia have an increased risk for PTSD and depression after childbirth. Therefore, after exploring their worries and fears, opting for caesarean section for women with this background can increase the satisfaction with childbirth and reduce this psychological morbidity.

3.2 Urinary incontinence

The EPICONT study observed 8.4% higher prevalence of urinary incontinence among women who had vaginal deliveries compared with those who had caesarean deliveries [37]. A study by Gyhagen et al. in 2013 found that the prevalence of urinary incontinence at more than 10 years after a single vaginal birth was 40.3% compared with 28.8% after one birth *via* caesarean section [38]. Nevertheless, National Institutes of Health consensus statement concluded that there was not enough evidence to recommend caesarean section for the sole prevention of urinary incontinence.

3.3 Pelvic organ prolapse

Up to 50% of all parous women have some degree of clinical prolapse and about 10–20% are symptomatic worldwide. Pregnancy and childbirth especially operative vaginal deliveries are known risk factors for pelvic organ prolapse (POP). A Swedish study found that the prevalence of symptomatic POP 20 years after one birth was doubled after a vaginal delivery compared with caesarean section [39].

3.4 Foetal complication

Foetal or newborn morbidity and mortality linked to labour and vaginal delivery are reduced or eliminated by caesarean birth. At the same time, intrapartum complications such as brachial plexus injury due to shoulder dystocia, bone trauma, and asphyxia related to intrapartum events may be prevented or avoided [9]. However, less than 10% of cerebral palsies are attributed to intrapartum events [40, 41]. Despite increasing rates of caesarean section, cerebral palsies rates have remained the same. Foetal neurological injuries affect 2–3% of births and are more common with operative vaginal deliveries. Current data suggest that the number of caesarean sections needed to prevent one cerebral palsy is 5000 and to prevent one permanent brachial plexus injury is 10000 [24]. Therefore, women should be counselled that elective caesarean section has no benefit in preventing cerebral palsy and brachial plexus injury. Nevertheless, the foetal outcome in terms of birth asphyxia, meconium stained liquor and need for Neonatal ICU admission are significantly higher in emergency caesarean section than in elective caesarean section [42].

3.5 Maternal morbidity

Vaginal delivery can be an unpredictable process even in a low-risk pregnancy. Situations such as foetal distress and poor progress of labour require emergency caesarean section, which carries an increased risk of morbidity compared with planned caesarean section. Post-operative wound infection, post-partum haemorrhage, need for blood transfusion, urinary tract infection, maternal pyrexia and need for intensive care unit admission are significantly higher in emergency caesarean section than elective caesarean section [42]. Limited data reporting showed that fatal injuries, including iatrogenic surgical injury, damage to the bladder or ureter, and pulmonary embolism seemed to be lower with planned CS than VD [9].

4. Ethical and medico-legal concerns

The infant is more likely to experience short- and long-term difficulties if a planned CS is performed on the mother's desire without a valid medical reason [35]. Over the past few years, numerous guidelines have emerged, including the one by NICE, issued in response to the discussion around the medical, ethical and financial effects of increased rates of caesarean sections on maternal request [43]. Given the considerable amount of uncertainty regarding the therapeutic benefits and risks of CSMR compared with vaginal birth, professional guidelines do not require addressing this option with every patient [9]. Even though the increases in absolute risk are frequently minimal, it may still be an unethical practice. Additionally, the fact that various maternity facilities and medical personnel might diversely respond to women's requests for C-sections may also lead to ethical dilemmas and healthcare inequities [35].

The choice of delivery frequently occurs based on the obstetrician's beliefs and experiences, the patient's gravidity, the hospital's environment and internal protocols, the rising prevalence of labour induction, the medico-legal implications and, finally, the mother's right to request a caesarean section without a doctor's recommendation [29]. An obstetrician's decision making and counselling may frequently be guided by the fear of litigation [38]. In obstetric practice, a lawsuit is a frequent occurrence that can be stressful for healthcare professionals, so they try to avoid legal action [29]. Worldwide, the number of lawsuits involving obstetric care is steadily increasing. Therefore, meticulous counselling and explanation about the risk versus benefits should be done on a case-to-case basis during the antenatal period.

5. Conclusion

The following chapter has comprehensively summarized the current clinical scenario of caesarean section on maternal request and highlighted some key points through a vigorous review of the literature. CS can be a promising surgical intervention in medically relevant cases but should be guided by ethically driven norms. Since data unavailability or lack of information on birth certificates/discharge sheets accounts for a major limitation in addressing the actual prevalence of CSMR, appropriate registries should be designed for reporting and recording patients seeking elective CS. Strategic measures should be implemented to identify and manage the determinants of CSMR (medical, psychological and psychosocial, social, cultural and economic) that may lead women to request CS delivery and thus contribute to the massive global economic impact.

Although CSMR has been linked to certain beneficial outcomes (e.g. reduced urinary incontinence and pelvic organ prolapse, reduced rate of PTSD and depression, and lesser intrapartum complications), it still imposes maternal (e.g. post-partum haemorrhage and infection, visceral damage, placenta accrete, placental abruption and complications in future pregnancy) and foetal (stillbirth, asphyxia, respiratory distress and other pulmonary infections) adverse outcomes as well. Since CS is associated with both short- and long-term health complications, it is essential to control the potential risk factors before proceeding with a planned C-section.

CS requests from the mother should be approved by informed consent, which pinpoints the complications, amplifies the absence of a clinical indication and provides necessary information about this absence. In conclusion, medical professionals should seek to provide women with the right advice, not to discourage them from having a caesarean delivery but, more importantly, to support them in having a positive birth experience. Future approaches and efforts should be directed toward mitigating clinically unrequired CS procedures due to medical malpractices, lack of awareness in women and the underlying determinants of elective CS that led to its widespread practices.

Acknowledgements

The authors would like to acknowledge all faculties and departments at the University of Malaya for their consistency in producing significant research.

Conflict of interest

The authors declare no conflict of interest.

DOI: http://dx.doi.org/10.5772/intechopen.109589

Author details

Neha Sethi*, Rajeev Kumar Rajaratnam and Nadiah Abdullah
Faculty of Medicine, Department of Obstetrics and Gynaecology, University of Malaya, Kuala Lumpur, Malaysia

*Address all correspondence to: s_neha26@um.edu.my

References

[1] Cunningham FG, Gant NF, Leveno KJ, Gilstrap LC III, Hauth JC, Wenstrom KD. Williams Obstetrics. 21st ed. New York: McGraw-Hill; 2001. p. 1668

[2] Teguete I, Traore Y, Sissoko A, Djire MY, Thera A, Dolo T, et al. Determining factors of cesarean delivery trends in developing countries: Lessons from point G National Hospital (Bamako-Mali). INTECH Open Access. 2012;**2012**:161-202

[3] American College of Obstetricians and Gynecologists. ACOG Committee Opinion No. 761: Cesarean Delivery on Maternal Request. Obstetrics Gynecology. 2019;**133**:e73

[4] Muhammad T, Srivastava S, Kumar P, Rashmi R. Prevalence and predictors of elective and emergency caesarean delivery among reproductive-aged women in Bangladesh: Evidence from demographic and health survey, 2017-18. BMC Pregnancy and Childbirth. 2022;**22**(1):1-1

[5] Harrison MS, Garces A, Figueroa L, Esamai F, Bucher S, Bose C, et al. Caesarean birth by maternal request: a poorly understood phenomenon in low-and middle-income countries. International Health. 2021;**13**(1):63-69

[6] American College of Obstetricians and Gynecologists. ACOG Committee Opinion No. 394: Cesarean Delivery on Maternal Request. Obstetrics and Gynecology. 2007;**110**:1501. DOI: 10.1097/01.AOG.0000291577.01569.4c

[7] Betrán AP, Ye J, Moller AB, Zhang J, Gülmezoglu AM, Torloni MR. The increasing trend in caesarean section rates: Global, regional and national estimates: 1990-2014. PLoS One. 2016;**11**(2):e0148343

[8] Norwitz ER. Birth, potential benefits of planned cesarean, and risks of planned cesarean birth. Cesarean Birth on Maternal Request. UpToDate. 2022;**2022**:6-9

[9] Gholitabar M, Ullman R, James D, Griffiths M. Caesarean section: Summary of updated NICE guidance. BMJ. 2011;**2011**:343. DOI: 10.1136/bmj.d7108

[10] Rahman M, Khan N, Rahman A, Alam M, Khan A. Long-term effects of caesarean delivery on health and behavioural outcomes of the mother and child in Bangladesh. Journal of Health, Population, and Nutrition. 2022;**41**(1):1-7

[11] Lumbiganon P, Laopaiboon M, Gulmezoglu AM, Souza JP, Taneepanichskul S, Pang RY, et al. Method of delivery and pregnancy outcomes in Asia: The WHO global survey on maternal and perinatal health 2007-08. Lancet. 2010;**375**(9713):490-499

[12] Potter JE, Hopkins K, Faúndes A, Perpétuo I. Women's autonomy and scheduled cesarean sections in Brazil: A cautionary tale. Birth. 2008;**35**:33-40

[13] Kovavisarach E, Ruttanapan K. Self-preferred route of delivery of thai obstetricians and gynecologists. Journal of the Medical Association of Thailand. 2016;**99**(Suppl. 2):S84-S90

[14] Deng R, Tang X, Liu J, Gao Y, Zhong X. Cesarean delivery on maternal request and its influencing factors in Chongqing, China. BMC Pregnancy and Childbirth. 2021;**21**(1):1-2. DOI: 10.1186/s12884-021-03866-7

[15] Karalasingam SD, Jeganathan R, Jegasothy R, Reidpath DD. Caesarean section rates from Malaysian tertiary hospitals using Robson's 10-group classification. BMC Pregnancy and Childbirth. 2020;**20**(1):1-8. DOI: 10.1186/s12884-020-2760-2

[16] Gruber J, Owings M. Physician financial incentives and cesarean section delivery. The RAND Journal of Economics. 1996;**27**(1):99-123. DOI: 10.2307/2555794

[17] Gibbons L, Belizán JM, Lauer JA, Betrán AP, Merialdi M, Althabe F. The global numbers and costs of additionally needed and unnecessary caesarean sections performed per year: Overuse as a barrier to universal coverage. World Health Report. 2010;**30**:1-31

[18] Haider MR, Rahman MM, Moinuddin M, Rahman AE, Ahmed S, Khan MM. Ever-increasing Caesarean section and its economic burden in Bangladesh. PLoS One. 2018;**13**(12):e0208623

[19] Parveen R, Khakwani M, Naz A, Bhatti R. Analysis of cesarean sections using Robson's Ten Group Classification System. Pakistan Journal of Medical Sciences. 2021;**37**(2):567. DOI: 10.12669/pjms.37.2.3823

[20] Liu S, Liston RM, Joseph KS, Heaman M, Sauve R, Kramer MS. Maternal mortality and severe morbidity associated with low-risk planned cesarean delivery versus planned vaginal delivery at term. CMAJ. 2007;**176**(4):455-460

[21] Masciullo L, Petruzziello L, Perrone G, Pecorini F, Remiddi C, Galoppi P, et al. Caesarean section on maternal request: An Italian comparative study on patients' characteristics, pregnancy outcomes and guidelines overview. International Journal of Environmental Research and Public Health. 2020;**17**(13):4665. DOI: 10.3390/ijerph17134665

[22] O'Connell MA, Leahy-Warren P, Khashan AS, Kenny LC, O'Neill SM. Worldwide prevalence of tocophobia in pregnant women: Systematic review and meta-analysis. Acta Obstetricia et Gynecologica Scandinavica. 2017;**96**:907-920

[23] Molgora S, Fenaroli V, Prino LE, Rollè L, Sechi C, Trovato A, et al. Fear of childbirth in primiparous Italian pregnant women: The role of anxiety, depression, and couple adjustment. Women and Birth. 2018;**31**(2):117-123

[24] Gnanasambanthan S, Datta S. When is a maternal request caesarean section not a maternal request? Obstetrics, Gynaecology and Reproductive Medicine. 2020;**30**(6):190-193. DOI: doi.org/10.1016/j.ogrm.2020.03.003

[25] Størksen HT, Garthus-Niegel S, Adams SS, Vangen S, Eberhard-Gran M. Fear of childbirth and elective caesarean section: A population-based study. BMC Pregnancy and Childbirth. 2015;**15**:221. DOI: 10.1186/s12884-015-0655-4

[26] Béhague DP, Victora CG, Barros FC. Consumer demand for caesarean sections in Brazil: Informed decision making, patient choice, or social inequality? A population based birth cohort study linking ethnographic and epidemiological methods. BMJ. 2002;**324**(7343):942

[27] Hsu KH, Liao PJ, Hwang CJ. Factors affecting Taiwanese women's choice of cesarean section. Social Science & Medicine. 2008;**66**(1):201-209

[28] Sorrentino F, Greco F, Palieri T, Vasciaveo L, Stabile G, Carlucci S, et al.

Caesarean section on maternal request-ethical and juridic issues: A narrative review. Medicina (Kaunas, Lithuania). 2022;**58**(9):1255. DOI: 10.3390/medicina58091255

[29] Sharpe AN, Waring GJ, Rees J, McGarry K, Hinshaw K. Caesarean section at maternal request—The differing views of patients and healthcare professionals: A questionnaire based study. European Journal of Obstetrics, Gynecology, and Reproductive Biology. 2015;**192**:54-60. DOI: 10.1016/j.ejogrb.2015.06.014

[30] McCourt C, Weaver J, Statham H, Beake S, Gamble J, Creedy DK. Elective cesarean section and decision making: A critical review of the literature. Birth. 2007;**34**(1):65-79

[31] O'donovan C, O'donovan J. Why do women request an elective cesarean delivery for non-medical reasons? A systematic review of the qualitative literature. Birth. 2018;**45**(2):109-119

[32] Abbaspoor Z, Moghaddam-Banaem L, Ahmadi F, Kazemnejad A. Iranian mothers' selection of a birth method in the context of perceived norms: A content analysis study. Midwifery. 2014;**30**(7):804-809

[33] Zhao Y, Chen S. Psychosocial factors for women requesting cesarean section. International Journal of Clinical Medicine. 2013;**4**(9):395

[34] Swedish Agency for Health Technology Assessment and Assessment of Social Services (SBU). Caesarean Section on Maternal Request: A Systematic Review and Assessment of Medical, Health Economic, Ethical and Social Aspects. Stockholm: Swedish Agency for Health Technology Assessment and Assessment of Social Services (SBU); 2021. Available from: https://www.ncbi.nlm.nih.gov/books/NBK580955/

[35] Keag OE, Norman JE, Stock SJ. Long-term risks and benefits associated with cesarean delivery for mother, baby, and subsequent pregnancies: Systematic review and meta-analysis. PLoS Medicine. 2018;**15**(1):e1002494

[36] D'Souza R. Caesarean section on maternal request for non-medical reasons: Putting the UK National Institute of Health and Clinical Excellence guidelines in perspective. Best Practice & Research. Clinical Obstetrics & Gynaecology. 2013;**27**(2):165-177

[37] Rortveit G, Daltveit AK, Hannestad YS, Hunskaar S, Norwegian EPINCONT Study. Urinary incontinence after vaginal delivery or cesarean section. The New England Journal of Medicine. 2003;**348**(10):900-907. DOI: 10.1056/NEJMoa021788

[38] Gyhagen M, Bullarbo M, Nielsen TF, Milsom I. The prevalence of urinary incontinence 20 years after childbirth: A national cohort study in singleton primiparae after vaginal or caesarean delivery. BJOG : An International Journal of Obstetrics and Gynaecology. 2013;**120**(2):144-151. DOI: 10.1111/j.1471-0528.2012.03301.x

[39] Gyhagen M, Bullarbo M, Nielsen TF, Milsom I. Prevalence and risk factors for pelvic organ prolapse 20 years after childbirth: A national cohort study in singleton primiparae after vaginal or caesarean delivery. BJOG. Jan 2013;**120**(2):152-160. DOI: 10.1111/1471-0528.12020. Epub 2012 Nov 2. PMID: 23121158

[40] Bakketeig LS. Only a minor part of cerebral palsy cases begin in labour. But still room for controversial childbirth issues in court. BMJ.

1999;**319**(7216):1016-1017. DOI: 10.1136/bmj.319.7216.1016

[41] Weil O, Fernandez H. Is safe motherhood an orphan initiative? The Lancet. 1999;**354**(9182):940-943

[42] Darnal N, Dangal G. Maternal and fetal outcome in emergency versus elective caesarean section. Journal of Nepal Health Research Council. 2020;**18**(2):186-189. DOI: 10.33314/jnhrc.v18i2.2093

[43] Capobianco G, Angioni S, Dessole M, Cherchi PL. Cesarean section: To be or not to be, is this the question? Archives of Gynecology and Obstetrics. 2013;**288**(2):461-462

Section 3

Cesarean Section in Teenagers, Old Women and Cesarean Section and Preterm Birth

Chapter 4

Cesarean Delivery and Mental Health

Evangelia Antoniou, Eirini Orovou, Alexandros Papatrechas, Christiana Arampatzi and Panagiotis Eskitzis

Abstract

A delivery by cesarean can be a cause of development of mental illness, especially posttraumatic stress disorder or the profile of the disorder for a percentage of women. Despite the global increase in cesarean deliveries, there is a paucity of adequate research into posttraumatic stress disorder after cesarean delivery and at many times is associated with other mental disorders of the postpartum period. The purpose of this research is to identify if there is a link between the type of cesarean delivery and posttraumatic stress disorder among postpartum women. Our sample consisted of 162 women who underwent a cesarean section in a public University Hospital in Greece and consented to participate in the study. The results show a high prevalence of postpartum posttraumatic stress disorder (31.7%) and profile postpartum posttraumatic stress disorder (14.3%) in women after emergency cesarean delivery with additional risk factors of preterm delivery, inclusion in Neonatal Intensive Care Unit, lack of support from the partner, and lack of breastfeeding.

Keywords: cesarean delivery, emergency cesarean section, elective cesarean section, posttraumatic stress disorder, postpartum period, mental health

1. Introduction

Posttraumatic stress disorder (PTSD) is a psychiatric disorder that may occur to a person who has experienced or witnessed a traumatic event such as a natural disaster, a serious accident, sexual violence, threatened death or death, serious injury, or extreme repeated exposure to the workplace [1]. PTSD has been known by other names in the past, such as "shell shock" during the World War I and "combat fatigue" after World War II. PTSD can happen in all people of any nationality or culture and at any age [2]. However, the prevalence of PTSD is about 10–12% in women and 5–6% in men [3], and this shows how it is influenced by traumatic birth experiences, hormonal disorders, stressful life events, and domestic violence [4]. PTSD is diagnosed after a month of a traumatic event and characterized by four main types of symptoms: re-experiencing, avoidance, negative thoughts and feelings, and arousal [5].

On the other hand, partial or profile PTSD involves many PTSD symptoms but not all, since persons exposed to the traumatic event do not meet all PTSD criteria. This is PTSD profile, which has been shown to be associated with high rates of suicidal ideation, alcoholism, absence in the working environment, and overconsumption of health services [6, 7].

1.1 Postpartum PTSD (P-PTSD)

For several years, the birth experience was considered by scientists as a positive experience for the woman. In recent years, however, research into birth trauma has increased interest, and it is now known that one out of three women had a stressful childbirth experience [8], while approximately 6% of women will develop acute PTSD and up to 16% clinically significant PTSD symptoms [9].

A traumatic birth experience can affect to a significant extend the woman herself and her family. Actually, P-PTSD may impair a mother-child bond and has an indirect adverse effect on the newborn's health. Also, P-PTSD or PTSD profile can overshadow the relationship with the partner and the desire to acquire another child in the future [10].

P-PTSD is the outcome of interaction between pre-labor, intrapartum, and postpartum vulnerability factors [11]. Various conditions seem to affect the development of this disorder, such as pregnancy pathology, complications during birth, emergency cesarean section, personal history of psychiatric disorders, fear of childbirth, and previous traumatic events in the mother's life [12–15]. Past traumatic life events may lead to a new PTSD after a traumatic birth experience. For explanation, the past traumas can be recalled and cause posttraumatic symptoms of an old PTSD [12, 13, 16].

Comorbidity of P-PTSD and depression is a very common phenomenon as evident in up to 70% of postpartum women endorsing P-PTSD [17]. Furthermore, suicidal ideation prevails in about 20% of women with P-PTSD [9], and for this reason, this postpartum mental disorder deserves more attention.

1.2 P-PTSD after cesarean delivery

The type of delivery and the P-PTSD was the subject of research by several researchers [10, 18, 19]. Regarding cesarean sections (CSs), however, there are studies that do not differentiate the outcome between emergency cesarean section (EMCS) and elective cesarean section (ELCS), and they finally consider that there is no connection between EMCS and PTSD [20–23]. On the other hand, there are many surveys that support a strong relationship between P-PTSD and EMCS in contrast to other kinds of delivery [16, 24–26]. So far, only two surveys investigate the correlation between EMCS and P-PTSD. A study published in 1997 was the first one showing that the majority of women experienced EMCS as a mental trauma [27], as well as a following article, that investigated the P-PTSD symptoms 3 months postpartum [27]. An explanation for this correlation is that the EMCS could be an unexpected outcome for some women who going through a difficult vaginal delivery were rushed into the operating room and underwent surgery with spinal/epidural anesthesia and in some cases, general anesthesia [28]. Furthermore, some studies also identified that past traumatic life events, low social support, poor coping skills, and psychiatric history are more determining factors for the development of P-PTSD [11, 13, 29].

1.3 P-PTSD after cesarean delivery in Greece

In Greece during 2019, there were about 85.000 [30], of which more than 50% were CS [31]. As a result, Greece occupies one of the greater positions worldwide [32].

DOI: http://dx.doi.org/10.5772/intechopen.108847

Apart from Greece, other countries such as Turkey, Mexico, Chile, Korea, Poland, and Hungary have been in the top positions in the world [33], which shows that the mothers of these countries are more exposed to birth trauma and consequently, more likely to develop P-PTSD or other mental disorder of postpartum period. So far, no research has been carried out in Greek women on P-PTSD or PTSD Profile, while the data are limited to other medical disorders of the postpartum period, such as depression [34, 35]. Therefore, this is the first survey that investigates P-PTSD in Greek women and specifically in a group of women who are more exposed to birth trauma. The purpose of this investigation is first to study the frequency of P-PTSD between two groups of women (EMCS and ELCS) in the sixth week postpartum and secondly to determine the risk factors and their degree of contribution to the development of P-PTSD and PTSD Profile. After identifying the risk factors, it is expected to develop specialized midwifery interventions and treatment in women with P-PTSD. This survey should signal the start of further investigations in the P-PTSD in Greece.

2. Methods

This prospective cohort study took place from July to November 2019, at the obstetric Clinic of the University Hospital of Larisa in Greece. The survey was approved by the Ethics Commission of Hospital. Approval: 18838/08-05-2019. This study used a descriptive design to record the prevalence of P-PTSD and PTSD Profile 6 weeks after CS (Criterion F of PTSD, DSM-5) [36]. As well as the risk factors that may lead to the development of these disorders.

2.1 Study participants

All participants were postpartum women who underwent a CS and had a medical dossier in the specific hospital. From this study excluded all women with issues at a cognitive level, who do not speak Greek or those whose pregnancy was monitored in another hospital. Furthermore, the women who used psychotropic substances or drugs were excluded (Criterion H of PTSD, DSM-5) [36], as well as underage mothers.

2.2 Data and measures

The data were collected in two stages. The first stage was the second day after CS, and the second stage was the sixth week after childbirth. During the first stage that coincides with the recovery of the woman after cesarean delivery, so that they can answer the questions of the psychometric tools, we collected medical, sociodemographic, past traumatic life events, and the identification or not of the cesarean delivery being a traumatic event from the total sample of 160 women who met the criteria for participation. The specific period of time was selected in order to meet the Criterion F of DSM-5 of PTSD [36]. All measures were made By the National Center of PTSD staff according to the DSM-5 Criteria [5] translated and weighted into the Greek language by the investigator midwife.

2.2.1 Sociodemographic questionnaire

The research-made questionnaire includes items on medical (obstetric/neonatal), social, demographic, and mental characteristics of the postpartum women. It also included information on the experience of the traumatic cesarean delivery or conditions associated with neonatal complications.

2.2.2 The life events checklist (LEC-5) of DSM-5

The LEC-5 is a self-report tool for screen previous traumatic events in a person's life. The measure evaluates exposure to 16 traumatic events known to result in trauma and one item evaluating any other event not captured in 16 items [37]. The LEC-5 is the only measure that the persons can define different exposure status of a traumatic event, while there is no score or rating [38].

2.2.3 Posttraumatic stress checklist (PCL-5) of DSM-V

The (PCL-5) is a self-report measure, authored by the National Center of PTSD according to the DSM-5, which was constructed to assess PTSD symptoms. In this study, the postpartum women answered via telephone to questions that corresponded to four groups of criteria (re-experiencing, avoidance, negative thoughts and feelings, arousal, and reactivity) [39]. The answers range by 0–4 and a score of 1 or more in items of re-experiencing and avoidance, and 2 or more in items of negative thoughts and feelings and arousal and reactivity, are considered as possible PTSD. If all the above criteria are met along with criterion A, the provisional diagnosis of PTSD is made. To diagnose the severity of the symptomatology, the score of the rating from all the answers can be used. A score $\geq$ 33 of PCL-5 can also considered as a possible PTSD [40–43]. The disorder is divided into two categories: (a) the provisional PTSD diagnosis and, (b) PTSD Profile (which includes some of its basic symptoms) [6, 7, 23]. The PCL-5 has very good psychometric properties and can be used to diagnose PTSD in many population groups [13, 44].

3. Results

Data from 160 postpartum women after EMCS and ELCS were analyzed. The sample characteristics according to the type of cesarean delivery are presented in **Table 1**. A percentage of 39.4% of women had an EMCS and 60.6% had an ELCS. Other demographic factors such as, age, nationality, family and financial status, and medical history are similar in the two groups of postpartum women. Women who underwent an ELCS were more likely to have a previous birth or a previous cesarean delivery and less likely to have a psychiatric history. Additionally, the median number of traumatic events that were recorded was greater in the group of women who had an EMCS.

3.1 Pregnancy and delivery characteristics

Pregnancy and delivery characteristics are shown in **Table 2**. In the EMCS group, a greater proportion of women had complications during pregnancy or required inclusion to the Neonatal Intensive Care Unit (NICU). Women with ELCS reported more support from their partners and had significantly lower proportions of reported traumatic birth experience. In addition, postpartum mothers with EMCS had a lower rate of breastfeeding (**Figure 1**) and expectations for their birth experience.

	Total sample (N = 160)	Type of c-section		P
		Emergency (N = 63; 39.4%)	Planned (N = 97; 60.6%)	
	N (%)	N (%)	N (%)	
Age, mean (SD)	33.1 (5.9)	32.7 (6.3)	33.4 (5.6)	0.506‡
Married/engaged/in a relationship	154 (96.3)	62 (98.4)	92 (94.8)	0.404++
Educational level				
Primary/middle/high school graduate	81 (50.6)	34 (54)	47 (48.5)	0.495+
University alumni/MSc/PhD	79 (49.4)	29 (46)	50 (51.5)	
Financial status				
Low	18 (11.3)	9 (14.3)	9 (9.3)	0.185++
Middle	134 (83.8)	53 (84.1)	81 (83.5)	
High	8 (5.0)	1 (1.6)	7 (7.2)	
Nationality				
Greek	149 (93.1)	57 (90.5)	92 (94.8)	0.344++
Other	11 (6.9)	6 (9.5)	5 (5.2)	
Parity				
0	79 (49.4)	46 (73)	33 (34)	<0.001+
1	61 (38.1)	13 (20.6)	48 (49.5)	
>1	20 (12.5)	4 (6.3)	16 (16.5)	
Type of previous labor				
Vaginal	16 (19.8)	8 (47.1)	8 (12.5)	0.010++
C-section	62 (76.5)	9 (52.9)	53 (82.8)	
Both	3 (3.7)	0 (0.0)	3 (4.7)	
Psychiatric history	21 (13.1)	8 (12.7)	8 (8.2)	0.337+
Number of traumatic events, median (IQR)	1 (0–2)	2 (0–4)	1 (0–3)	0.012‡‡
Medical history	54 (33.8)	23 (36.5)	31 (32)	0.552+

+*Pearson's chi-square test.*
++*Fisher's exact test.*
‡*Student's t-test.*
‡‡*Mann-Whitney test.*

Table 1.
Sample characteristics in total and according to the type of cesarean delivery.

3.2 The prevalence of PTSD symptoms among postpartum women

The prevalence of PTSD with Profile PTSD was 14.3% in women with EMCS and 4.1% in women with ELCS, while the prevalence of PTSD in women with EMCS was 31.7% and 1% in women with ELCS (**Figure 2**).

	Total sample (N = 160)	Type of CS		P
		EMCS (N = 63; 39.4%)	ELCS (N = 97; 60.6%)	
	N (%)	N (%)	N (%)	
Conception				
Normal	145 (90.6)	58 (92.1)	87 (89.7)	0.615⁺
IVF	15 (9.4)	5 (7.9)	10 (10.3)	
Problems during pregnancy	70 (43.8)	35 (55.6)	35 (36.1)	0.015⁺
Gestational week, mean (SD)	37.7 (2.1)	37.4 (3)	38 (1.2)	0.066‡
Preterm labor	133 (83.1)	48 (76.2)	85 (87.6)	0.059⁺
NICU	30 (18.8)	19 (30.2)	11 (11.3)	0.003⁺
Support from spouse	132 (82.5)	46 (73)	86 (88.7)	0.011⁺
Expectations	89 (55.6)	16 (25.4)	73 (75.3)	<0.001⁺
Traumatic c-section	64 (40)	45 (71.4)	19 (19.6)	<0.001⁺
Breastfeeding	110 (68.8)	36 (57.1)	74 (76.3)	0.011⁺

+*Pearson's chi-square test.*
‡*Student's t-test.*

Table 2.
Pregnancy and delivery characteristics.

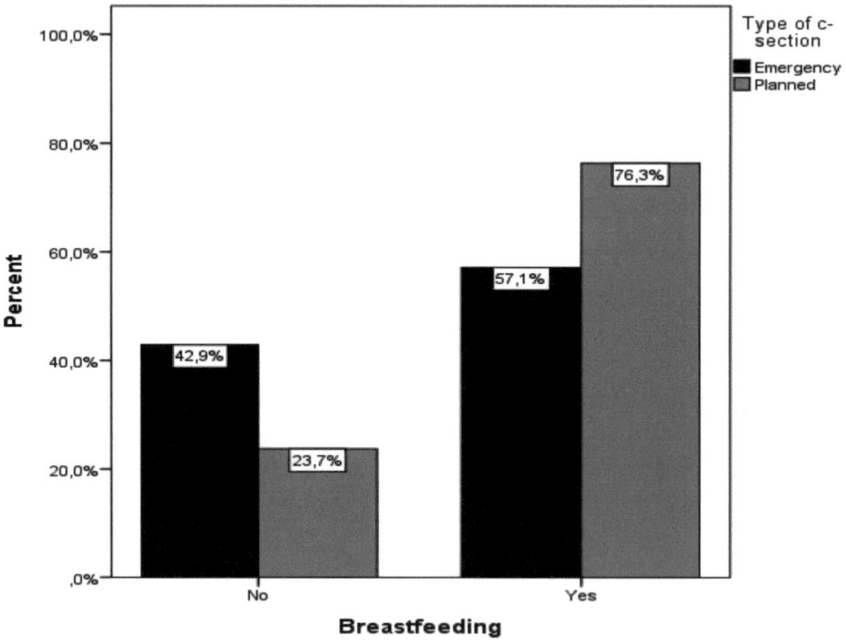

Figure 1.
Type of CS and rates of breastfeeding.

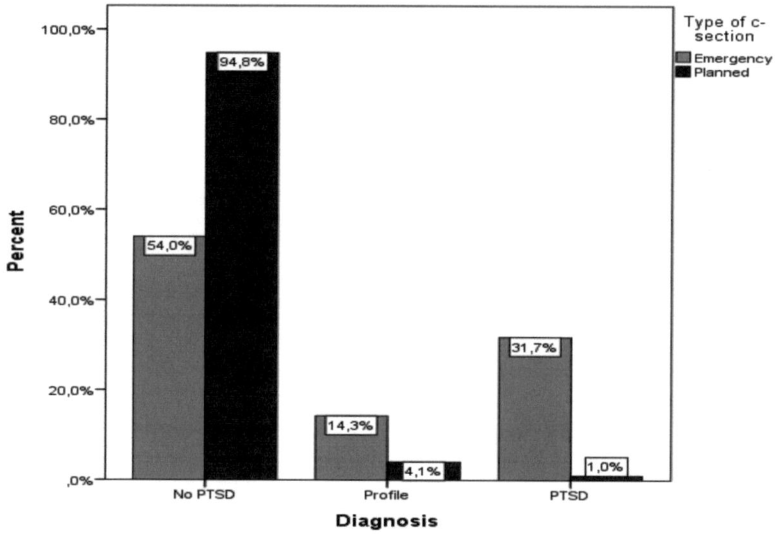

Figure 2.
Proportions of women with PTSD according to type of cesarean delivery.

Table 3 shows an overview of PTSD profile and PTSD symptoms in women after EMCS and ELCS. Among the postpartum women, the prevalence of criterion A is 25.6% (ELCS = 7.2% and EMCS = 54%) and those who met the other four criteria of symptoms is between 19 and 26.3% (ELCS = 7.2–10.3% and EMCS = 36.4–52.5%). After cesarean delivery, a total of 13.1% of women after CS met the all PTSD criteria according to the DSM-5.

	Total sample (N = 160)	Type of CS		P
		EMCS (N = 63; 39.4%)	ELCS (N = 97; 60.6%)	
	N (%)	N (%)	N (%)	
Criterion A	41 (25.6)	34 (54)	7 (7.2)	<0.001⁺
Re-experiencing (B)	42 (26.3)	33 (52.4)	9 (9.3)	<0.001⁺
Avoidance (C)	42 (26.3)	32 (50.8)	10 (10.3)	<0.001⁺
Negative thoughts and feelings (D)	43 (26.9)	33 (52.4)	10 (10.3)	<0.001⁺
Arousal and reactivity (E)	31 (19.4)	23 (36.5)	8 (8.2)	<0.001⁺
Diagnosis				
No PTSD	126 (78.8)	34 (54)	92 (94.8)	<0.001⁺
PTSD Profile	13 (8.1)	9 (14.3)	4 (4.1)	
Provisional PTSD	21 (13.1)	20 (31.7)	1 (1.0)	
PTSD score, median (IQR)	2 (0–17)	17 (2–32)	0 (0–4)	<0.001‡‡

⁺*Pearson's chi-square test.*
‡‡*Mann-Whitney test.*

Table 3.
PTSD profile and PTSD symptoms in women after EMCS and ELCS.

		Diagnosis		Unadjusted OR (95% CI)	P	Adjusted OR (95% CI)	P
		No PTSD/ Profile	PTSD				
		N (%)	N (%)				
Age		33.3 (5.7)	32 (7.3)	0.97 (0.90–1.04)	0.380	0.89 (0.77–1.03)	0.105
Married/ engaged/in a relationship	No	5 (83.3)	1 (16.7)	1.00[+]		1.00	
	Yes	134 (87.0)	20 (13.0)	0.75 (0.08–6.72)	0.794	0.53 (0.01–54.52)	0.787
Educational level	Primary/ middle/ high school graduate	70 (86.4)	11 (13.6)	1.00		1.00	
	University alumni/ MSc/PhD	69 (87.3)	10 (12.7)	0.92 (0.37–2.31)	0.863	1.43 (0.33–6.13)	0.630
Financial status	Low	14 (77.8)	4 (22.2)	1.00		1.00	
	Middle/ high	125 (88.0)	17 (12.0)	0.48 (0.14–1.61)	0.234	2.26 (0.16–32.05)	0.548
Nationality	Greek	129 (86.6)	20 (13.4)	1.00		1.00	
	Other	10 (90.9)	1 (9.1)	0.65 (0.08–5.31)	0.684	0.16 (0.01–3.11)	0.225
Parity	0	66 (83.5)	13 (16.5)	1.00		1.00	
	> = 1	73 (90.1)	8 (9.9)	0.56 (0.22–1.43)	0.222	1.36 (0.11–16.79)	0.810
Previous CS	No	79 (83.2)	16 (16.8)	1.00		1.00	
	Yes	60 (92.3)	5 (7.7)	0.41 (0.14–1.19)	0.100	0.9 (0.05–15.07)	0.944
Psychiatric history	No	126 (90.6)	13 (9.4)	1.00		1.00	
	Yes	13 (61.9)	8 (38.1)	5.96 (2.09–17.04)	0.001	2.79 (0.55–14.17)	0.216
Number of traumatic events, median (IQR)		1 (0–3)	3 (1–5)	1.29 (1.06–1.57)	0.013	1.34 (0.84–2.18)	0.211
Full-term labor	No	18 (66.7)	9 (33.3)	1.00		1.00	
	Yes	121 (91)	12 (9)	0.19 (0.07–0.54)	0.001	0.34 (0.06–1.83)	0.208

		Diagnosis		Unadjusted OR (95% CI)	P	Adjusted OR (95% CI)	P
		No PTSD/ Profile	PTSD				
		N (%)	N (%)				
Type of CS	Planned	96 (99.0)	1 (1.0)	1.00		1.00	
	Emergency	43 (68.3)	20 (31.7)	44.65 (5.80–343.50)	<0.001	46.55 (6.00–360.81)	<0.001
NICU	No	121 (93.1)	9 (6.9)	1.00		1.00	
	Yes	18 (60.0)	12 (40)	8.96 (3.31–24.27)	<0.001	9.00 (3.31–24.49)	<0.001
Support from partner	No	20 (71.4)	8 (28.6)	1.00		1.00	
	Yes	119 (90.2)	13 (9.8)	0.27 (0.10–0.74)	0.011	0.27 (0.10–0.74)	0.011
Expectations	No	50 (70.4)	21 (29.6)				
	Yes	89 (100.0)	0 (0.0)	–++	—	—	—
Traumatic CS	No	96 (100.0)	0 (0.0)				
	Yes	43 (67.2)	21 (32.8)	–++	—	—	—
Breastfeeding	No	34 (68.0)	16 (32.0)	1.00		1.00	
	Yes	105 (95.5)	5 (4.5)	0.10 (0.03–0.30)	<0.001	0.08 (0.02–0.25)	<0.001

+*Pearson's chi-square test.*
++*Fisher's exact test.*

Table 4.
Risk factors for PTSD after cesarean delivery.

3.3 Risk factors for PTSD after cesarean delivery

According to the univariate regression analyses with dependent variable as the presence of postpartum PTSD (**Table 4**) presented a positive association between psychiatric history, inclusion in NICU, EMCS, and number of past traumatic events with the likelihood of PTSD diagnosis. Women, who breastfed, those with full-term labor, and those who reported having support from their partner, had lower likelihood of having postpartum PTSD. In **Table 4**, multiple analyses reveal that the type of cesarean delivery is independently linked with postpartum PTSD after cesarean delivery.

4. Discussion

The aim of this survey was to identify perinatal and predisposing factors during cesarean delivery that help the development of PTSD or PTSD Profile in postpartum period, in order to realize appropriate preventive interventions in perinatal care. Our findings show that 40% of mothers reported their cesarean delivery as a traumatic event, while the Criterion A met by a quarter of all deliveries. Moreover, we found that postpartum PTSD was associated with preterm birth, inclusion in NICU, lack of breastfeeding, EMCS, and lack of support from a partner.

Several previous studies were considered the emergency cesarean delivery as a major risk factor for postpartum mental illness, such as depression [45–47] and PTSD [27, 48]. For example, the Schwab et al. study shows that all women who had been diagnosed with postpartum PTSD had undergone an EMCS [16]. The systematic review of Benton et al. found an association between EMCS and psychological outcomes in mothers with particular postpartum PTSD [49]. In addition, the Modaress et al. study found high levels of PTSD in women who underwent an EMCS in contrast to ELCS and those with vaginal delivery [50]. Furthermore, the findings of Ryding et al. investigation for PTSD reaction in women who underwent an EMCS showed that 1/3 of the sample suffered from serious PTSD reactions [48]. On the contrary, the study by Lopez et al. found no association between PTSD and a kind of CS, but with anesthesia complications [23]. Also, a systematic review of Futura et al. found a relationship with preeclampsia, rather than the type of CS [51].

However, the present study found that 13.1% of the population met the DSM-5 criteria for postpartum PTSD (31.7% after EMCS and 1% after ELCS), while 8.1% of women were suffering from Profile PTSD according to DSM-5 (**Table 3**). A possible explanation for the high difference in prevalence among two groups of mothers is due to the emergency surgery. Since, emergency surgery is unexpected more often with the pathology of gestation [50, 52], and can be a midwifery predictor of the development of postpartum PTSD [8, 27]. Therefore, the increase in EMCS increase PTSD, while an important reason for this phenomenon might be that the induction of labor takes place before the 41st week of gestation [53, 54].

An observation must be made regarding ours and other research findings. This survey is the first to investigate the evolvement of PTSD Profile and PTSD in postpartum women after EMCS or ELCS. In addition, it is one of the few articles where they used all the diagnostic criteria for PTSD postpartum, according to the DSM-5 (**Table 3**) [13], and this increases the sensitivity of the PCL-5 compared with common investigations in the past. So far, the fifth version of the PCL has not been in used in Greece yet. This is the first survey that used the PCL-5 in the Greek population and especially in postpartum women.

The findings of our study indicated that a preterm labor is associated with PTSD. From the survey participants, only 76.2% women after EMCS and 87.6% after ELCS had a full-term labor, and 1/3 of women who met the diagnostic criteria for PTSD or PTSD Profile had given birth prematurely. Only a few studies in the past have reported that a preterm delivery was a risk factor for PPTSD and other postpartum mental health disorders [55–57], and our study agrees with them. One hypothesis is that prematurity is related to emergency situations, neonatal complications, and inclusion in the NICU. Therefore, the risk of losing an infants' life is real (the adapted for the present research criterion A) and the cause of the development of postpartum mental health trauma.

In addition, another very important risk factor related to the previous one for the development of postpartum PTSD is the inclusion of the neonate in the NICU. It seems that the separation of the mother from the infant due to the admission to NICU is associated with a birth of a preterm neonate, pathology of gestation, and EMCS as well. It is already known that the postpartum distress after the admission of the neonate in the NICU consists of a complication of depressive, anxiety, and PTSD symptoms and is linked negatively with maternal-infant attachment [56, 58]. In our findings, inclusion in the NICU is related to 11.3% of ELCS and 30.2% of EMCS and includes preterm and full-term neonates.

For a large percentage of women, breastfeeding is an extension of the birth experience, and it has been proven that it can reduce the birth trauma. In some cases, breastfeeding after a traumatic childbirth experience can be disappointing due to traumatic reminders of childbirth. All these feelings, as a part of avoidance symptoms of PTSD (Criterion C) [36], can lead to a lack of initiation or premature termination of breastfeeding [59]. In this survey, the lack of breastfeeding played an important role in the development of the birth trauma caused to the woman by the cesarean delivery, with rates of 95% in the first 24 h breastfeeding mothers without PTSD and 4.5% in breastfeeding mothers with PTSD. Therefore, breastfeeding is a relief by increasing the mental resistance of mothers exposed to birth trauma. These results are similar with the Hoff et al. study, which investigates that the lack of breastfeeding affects the development of the mother-child attachment and contributes to the intensity of the distress of the mother and developing postpartum PTSD [60]. Actually, in the Maureen et al. study, breastfeeding mothers had a lower perceived stress, lower depression and anger, and reported more positive life events than from postnatal PTSD [61–63].

Unfortunately, in Greece, there are few psychoeducation supporting services for women exposed to birth trauma. Among the few perinatal centers, Fainareti [64] is the first public perinatal center, which provides psychoeducation to mothers and couples. Due to this great lack of perinatal centers, support from a partner or spouse is one of the main factors protecting from postnatal PTSD.

5. Conclusions

The present research evaluated vulnerability postpartum risk factors in Greek mothers who had an EMCS or ELCS in a University Hospital. Birth trauma experience was predictive with the PCL-5 for cesarean deliveries. The measure revised to reflect the new diagnostic demands and now is one of the few validated tools for PTSD. Mothers in this survey who met all the diagnostic criteria (re-experiencing, avoidance, negative thoughts and feelings, arousal, and reactivity) of DSM-5 may have a provisional diagnosis of postpartum PTSD or PTSD Profile. Direct exposure and witnesses to birth trauma were predictive with the adapted Criterion A for postpartum women after cesarean delivery. From this study, it has emerged that the major risk factors developing postpartum PTSD are: inclusion in the NICU, preterm birth, EMCS, a lack of breastfeeding, and a lack of support from a partner. Perinatal health professionals who are in contact with women during pregnancy or postpartum should inform them in order to reduce the above risk factors. However, more research needs to be conducted with the aim of identifying more risk factors and reducing the rates of PTSD OR PTSD Profile, especially in countries similar to Greece with high percentages of CS. Finally, it should be understood by healthcare providers and health policymakers that the postpartum mental disorders are only a part of short-term and long-term negative effects of cesarean deliveries worldwide.

Acknowledgements

The authors would like to thank The Laboratory of Midwifery Care during Antenatal and Post natal period—Breastfeeding—L.M.C.A.P. – BF. of the University of West Attica.

Funding

From The Special Account for Research Grants, University of West Attica, Greece.

Conflict of interest

The authors declare no conflict of interest.

Author details

Evangelia Antoniou[1*], Eirini Orovou[1,2], Alexandros Papatrechas[3], Christiana Arampatzi[2] and Panagiotis Eskitzis[2]

1 Department of Midwifery, University of West Attica, Athens, Greece

2 Department of Midwifery, University of Western Macedonia, Ptolemaida, Greece

3 Faculty of Medicine, National and Kapodistrian University of Athens, Greece

*Address all correspondence to: lilanton@uniwa.gr

References

[1] PTSD. National Center for PTSD Home. Available from: https://www.ptsd.va.gov/index.asp. [Accessed: June 2020]

[2] What Is PTSD? Available from: https://www.psychiatry.orgjpatients·families/ptsd/what·is·ptsd. [Accessed: December 26, 2020]

[3] Olff M. Sex and gender differences in post·traumatic stress disorder: An update. Psychotraumatology. 2017;**8**(4):1351204

[4] Stein MB, Jang K. Genetic and environmental influences on trauma exposure and posttraumatic stress disorder symptoms: A twin study. American Journal of Psychiatry. 2002;**159**(10):1675-1681

[5] APA. DSM·5 diagnostic classification. In: Diagnostic and Statistical Manual of Mental Disorders; DSM Library. U.S.A: American Psychiatric Association; 2013

[6] Maes M. Partial posttraumatic stress disorder revisited. Affect Disorders. 2004;**78**(1):37-48

[7] Breslau N et al. Partial PTSD versus full PTSD: An empirical examination of associated impairment. Psychological Medicine. 2004;**34**(7):1205-1214

[8] Creedy DK, Shochet IM. Childbirth and the development of acute trauma symptoms: Incidence and contributing factors. Birth Berkeley. 2000;**27**(2):104-111

[9] Dekel S, Stuebe C, Dishy G. Childbirth induced posttraumatic stress syndrome: A systematic review of prevalence and risk factors. Frontiers in Psychology. 2017;**2017**:8

[10] Shaban Z, Dolatian M, Shams J, Alavi-Majd H, Mahmoodi Z, Sajjadi H. Post-traumatic stress disorder (PTSD) following childbirth: Prevalence and contributing factors. Iranium Red Crescent Medical 1.2013, 15 (3), 177-182

[11] Ayers S, Bond R, Bertullies S, Wijma K. The aetiology of PostTraumatic stress following childbirth: A meta-analysis and theoretical framework. Psychological Medicine. 2016;**46**(6):1121-1134

[12] Sentilhes L, Maillard F, Brun S, Madar H, Merlot B, Goffinet F, et al. Risk factors for chronic post-traumatic stress disorder development one year after vaginal delivery: A prospective, observational study. Scientific Reports. 2017;**7**(1):8724

[13] van Heumen MA, Hollander MH, van Pampus MG, van Dill en, 1; Stramrood, C. A. I. Psychosocial predictors of postpartum posttraumatic stress disorder in women with a traumatic childbirth experience. Frontiers in Psychiatry. 2018;**2018**:9

[14] Kessler RC, Sonnega A, Bromet E, Hughes M, Nelson CB. Posttraumatic stress disorder in the National Comorbidity Survey. Achieves in General Psychiatry. 1995;**52**(12):1048

[15] James S. Women's experiences of symptoms of posttraumatic stress disorder (PT SO) after traumatic childbirth: A review and critical appraisal. Achieves in Womens Mental Health. 2018;**18**(6):761

[16] Schwab W, Marth C, Bergant AM. Post-traumatic stress disorder post partum: The impact of birth on the prevalence of post-traumatic stress disorder (PTSD) in multiparous women. Geburtshilje Frauenheilkd. 2012;**72**(*1*):56-63

[17] Vildiz P, Ayers S, Phillips L. The prevalence of posttraumatic stress disorder in pregnancy and after birth: A systematic review and meta analysis. Affect Disorders. 2017;**208**:634-645

[18] Andersen LB, Melvaer LB, Videbech P, Lamont RF, Joergensen JS. Risk factors for developing post-traumatic stress disorder following childbirth: A systematic review. Acta Obstetrics Gynecology Scandinavian. 2012;**91**(11):1261-1272

[19] Mahmoodi Z, Dolatian M, Shaban Z, Shams L, Alavi-Ma H, Mirabzadeh A. Correlation between kind of delivery and posttraumatic stress disorder. Annals of Medicine. 2016;**6**(6):356-361

[20] Cohen MM et al. Posttraumatic stress disorder after pregnancy, labor, and delivery. Journal of Womens Health. 2004;**13**(3):315-324

[21] Sorenson DS, Tschetter L. Prevalence of negative birth perception, disaffirmation, perinatal trauma symptoms, and depression among postpartum women. Perspective Psychiatry. 2010;**46**(1):14-25

[22] Ford E, Ayers S, Bradley R. Exploration of a cognitive model to predict post-traumatic stress symptoms following childbirth. Anxiety Disorders. 2010;**24**(3):353-359

[23] Lopez U, Meyer M, Loures V, Iselin-Chaves I, Epiney M, Kern C, et al. Post-traumatic stress disorder in parturients delivering by caesarean section and the implication of anaesthesia: A Prospective Cohort Study. Health Quality Life Outcomes. 2017;**15**:692

[24] Czarnocka J, Slade P. Prevalence and predictors of post-traumatic stress symptoms following childbirth. Brazil Journal of Psychology. 2000;**39**(1):35-51

[25] Soderquist J, Wijma B, Thorbert G, Wijma K. Risk factors in pregnancy for post-traumatic stress and depression after childbirth. BJOG. 2009;**116**(5):672-680

[26] Garthus-Niegel S, von Soest T, Knoph C, Simonsen TB, Torgersen L, Eberhard-Gran M. The influence of women's preferences and actual mode of delivery on post-traumatic stress symptoms following childbirth: A population-based, longitudinal study. BMC Pregnancy Childbirth. 2014;**14**(1):191

[27] Tham V, Christensson K, Ryding E. Seme of coherence and symptoms of post-traumatic stress after emergency caesarean section. Acta Obstetricia et Gynecologica Scandinavica. 2007;**86**(9):1090-1096

[28] What is Birth Trauma?—Birth Trauma Association https://www.birthtraumaassociation.org.uk/for-parents/what-is-birthtraumail. [Accessed: January 3, 2021]

[29] O'Donovan A, Alcorn K, Patrick C, Creedy DK, Dawe S, Devilly G. Predicting posttraumatic stress disorder after childbirth. Midwi. 2014;**30**(8):935-941

[30] Statistics—ELSTAT. Available from: https://www.statistics.gr/en/statistics/-/publication/SP003/-. [Accessed: January 10, 2021]

[31] Antoniou E, Orovou E, Sarella A, et al. Is primary cesarean section a cause of increasing cesarean section rates in Greece? Material Sodo Medica. 2020;**32**(4):287

[32] WHO I Caesarean sections should only be performed when medically necessary says WHO. Available from: http://www.who.int/reproductivehealth/topics/maternal_perinatal/cs_statement/en/. [Accessed: January 10, 2021]

[33] Caesarean sections I Health at a Glance 2019: OECD Indicators I OECD i library. Available from: https://www.oecd-ilibrary.org/sites/fa1f7281-en/index.html?itemld=/content/component/fa1f7281-en. [Accessed: January 10, 2021]

[34] Leonardou AA et al. Validation of the Edinburgh postnatal depression scale and prevalence of postnatal depression at two months postpartum in a sample of Greek mothers. Reproduction in Psychology. 2009;**27**(1):28-39

[35] Papamarkou M, Sarafis P, Kaite CP, Tsounis A, Niakas D. Investigation of the association between quality of life and depressive symptoms during postpartum period: A correlational study. BMC Womens Health. 2017;**17**(1):115

[36] Treatment (US), c. for S. A. Exhibit 1.3-4, DSM-5 Diagnostic Criteria for PTSD. Available from: https://www.ncbLnlm.nih.gov/booksjNBK207191/. [Accessed: December 29, 2020]

[37] Life Events Checklist for DSM-5 (LEC-5)—PTSD: National Center for PTSD. Available from: https://www.ptsd.va.gov/professiona1/assessment/temeasures/life_events_checklist.asp. [Accessed: March 6, 2020]

[38] Gray M et al. Psychometric properties of the life events checklist. Assessment. 2004;**11**(4):330

[39] PTSD and DSM-5: unintended consequences of change. Available from: https://www.thelancet.com/;ournaIs/lanpsy/article/PIIS2215-0366(14)70321-9/fulltext. [Accessed: January 16, 2021]

[40] PTSO Checklist for OSM-5 (PCL-5)—PTSO: National Center for PTSO. https://www.ptsd.va.gov/professiona1/assessment/adult-sr/ptsdchecklist.asp. [Accessed: March 6, 2020]

[41] Greinacher A, Nikendei A, Kottke R. Secondary traumatization, psychological stress, and resilience in psychosocial emergency care personnel. Environmental Research Public Health. 2019;**16**(17):213

[42] Wortmann H, Jordan AH, et al. Psychometric analysis of the PTSD Checklist-5 (PCl –5) among treatment-seeking military service members. Psychological Assessment. 2016;**28**(11):1392-1403

[43] Blevins CA, Weathers FW, Davis MT, Witte TK. Domino,1l. The posttraumatic stress disorder checklist for DSM-5 (PCl –5): Development and initial psychometric Evaluation. Journal of Trauma. 2015;**28**(6):489-498

[44] Ayers S, Wright DB, Thornton A. Development of a measure of postpartum PTSD: The City birth trauma scale. Frontiers in Psychiatry. 2018;**2018**:9

[45] Xie R et al. Cesarean section and postpartum depression in a Cohort of Chinese Women with a High Cesarean Delivery Rate. Womens Health. 2022;**20**(12):1881-1886

[46] Boyee PM, Todd A. Increased risk of postnatal depression after emergency caesarean section. Medical Austrobaileya. 1992;**157**(3):172-174

[47] Ryding E, Wijma K, Wijma B. Psychological impact of emergency cesarean section in comparison with elective cesarean section, instrumental and normal vaginal delivery. Journal of Psychoses in Obstetrics and Gynaecology. 1998;**19**(3):135-144

[48] Ryding E, Wijma B, Wijma K. Posttraumatic stress reactions after emergency Cesarean section. Acta Obstetricia et Gynecologica Scandinavica. 1997;**76**(9):856-861

[49] Benton M, Salter A, Tape N, et al. Women's psychosocial outcomes following an emergency caesarean section: A systematic literature review. BMC Pregnancy Childbirth. 2019;**19**(1):535

[50] Modarres M, Afrasiabi S, Rahnama P, Montazeri A. Prevalence and risk factors of childbirth-related post-traumatic stress symptoms. BMC Pregnancy Childbirth. 2012;**12**(1):88

[51] Furuta M, Sand all, 1; Bick, D. A systematic review of the relationship between severe maternal morbidity and post-traumatic stress disorder. BMC Pregnancy Childbirth. 2012;**12**(1):125

[52] Karlstrom A. Women's self-reported experience of unplanned caesarean section: Results of a Swedish study. Midwifery. 2017;**50**:253-258

[53] Gayer I, Frank Wolf M. Induction of labor at 39 week5 of gestation versus expectant management. Hare. 2019;**158**(12):802

[54] World Health Organization. World Health Organization; World Health Organization Reproductive Health and Research. WHO; 2011

[55] Holditch-Davis O, Bartlett TR, Blickman A, Miles MS. Posttraumatic stress symptoms in mothers of premature infants. Journal of Obstetric, Gynecologic, and Neonatal Nursing. 2003;**32**(2):161-171

[56] Shaw R et al. Prevention of postpartum traumatic stress in mothers with preterm infants: Manual development and evaluation. Issues Mental Health Nursing. 2013;**34**(8):578-586

[57] Bonacquisti A, Geller PA, Patterson CA. Maternal depression, anxiety, stress, and maternal-infant attachment in the neonatal lntensive care unit. Journal of Reproduction. 2020;**38**(3):297-310

[58] Staver MA, Moore TA, Hanna KM, Harris-Haman PA, Zukowsky K. Maternal distress in the neonatal lntensive care unit: A concept analysis. Advanced in Neonatal Care. 2019;**19**(5):394-401

[59] Klein M, Vanderbilt O, Kendall-Tackett K. PTSD and breastfeeding: Let it flow. Nutrition. 2014;**6**(4):211-215

[60] Hoff CE, Mowa N, Rosen Vollmar AK, Perez-Escamilla R. Impact of maternal anxiety on breastfeeding outcomes: A systematic review. Advanced Nutrition. 2019;**10**(5):816-826

[61] Groi'k MW. Differences between exclusive breastfeeders, formulafeeders, and controls: A study of stress, mood, and endocrine variables. Bioscience Research Nursing. 2008;**7**(2):106-117

[62] Berkman F. The role of social relations in health promotion. psychosomatic Medicine. 1998;**57**(3):245-254

[63] Mayers A, Hambidge S, Bryant O, Arden-Close E. Supporting women who develop poor postnatal mental health: What support 00 fathers receive to support their partner and their own mental health? BMC Pregnancy Childbirth. 2020;**20**(1):359

[64] Perinatal care & support—fainareti. Available from: https://www.fainaretLgr/en/. [Accessed: October 21, 2020]

Section 4

Cesarean Section and Pregnancies Complicated by Thrombophilia, Antiphospholipid Syndrome and Congenital Heart Disease

Chapter 5

Difficult Cesarean Delivery

Awol Yemane Legesse and Hale Teka

Abstract

Cesarean section rate has been on the rise. It is commonly perceived as a simple and safe alternative to difficult vaginal birth. However, there are situations during C section where delivery of fetus may be difficult. There are multiple reasons for a cesarean section to be difficult such as poorly accessible lower segment, difficult fetal extraction, abnormal placentation, and visceral injuries. If the difficult cesarean section is not handled properly, it is high likely that the procedure will end up in catastrophic maternal and neonatal outcome. To avoid such disaster, it is imperative to have sufficient knowledge on anticipation, planning, and appropriate conduct of the procedure. Thus, this chapter aims at guiding practitioners on the management of common causes of difficult cesarean section.

Keywords: difficult CD, complicated CD, extensive adhesion, transverse lie, uterine incision

1. Introduction

Cesarean section (CS), defined as the birth of fetus through a surgical incision on the abdomen and uterine wall to effect delivery of fetus and product of conceptus, and it is one of the commonest obstetrical surgical procedures worldwide [1].

Cesarean section rate has been on the rise. It is commonly perceived as a simple and safe alternative to difficult vaginal birth. However, there are situations during C section where delivery of fetus may be difficult. There are multiple reasons for a cesarean section to be difficult such as poorly accessible lower segment, difficult fetal extraction, abnormal placentation, and visceral injuries [2].

If the difficult cesarean section is not handled properly, it is high likely that the procedure will end up in catastrophic maternal and neonatal outcome. To avoid such disaster, it is imperative to have sufficient knowledge on anticipation, planning, and appropriate conduct of the procedure [3].

Thus, this chapter aims at guiding practitioners on the management of common causes of difficult cesarean section.

To avoid such mishaps, anticipation of potential difficulties and planning in advance can be fruitful.

Before prepping and drapping the patient:

- Check the presenting part
- Check the location of the placenta

- Type of scar if she had previous scars
- Gestational age

2. Maternal and fetal factors contributing for difficult cesarean delivery

Absence of lower uterine segment, placenta previa, previous surgery with extensive adhesions, fibrous uterus are maternal factors which contribute for difficult cesarean delivery. Transverse lie, breech presentation, multiple pregnancy, small fetus are fetal factors commonly encountered in difficult cesarean section [3–5].

3. Classical uterine incision

Classical uterine incision is type of uterine incision in which the incision is made in the contractile part of the uterus so that the inaccessible lower segment can be bypassed. This is incision is usually deferred because it is susceptible to rupture with succeeding pregnancies. Most of the indications arise from difficulty in exposing the lower segment. In the remaining occasions, fetal indications such as transverse lie, and conjoined fetus dictate the incision [3].

3.1 Existing indications for classical CS

1. If the lower segment is not well developed and if intrauterine non routine maneuvers are anticipated
2. If there is tumor previa which poses difficulty for a transverse incision. (eg. large fibroid, anterior placenta previa)
3. Extensive bladder adhesion from previous repeat surgery.
4. Postmortem delivery
5. Transverse lie with the fetal back presenting over the pelvis
6. Leiomyoma filling the lower uterine segment
7. If cesarean hysterectomy is preplanned
8. If the previous classical section scar is highly thinned out
9. Cervix invaded by cancer

3.2 Surgical steps and technique

As with all surgery, lucid understanding of the anatomy is fundamental. The following listed techniques are to be followed during conduct of classical cesarean section.

3.3 Abdominal entry

1. Midline subumblical incision preferred

2. Open peritoneum in the upper part of the incision

3. Check that the uterus is not rotated

3.4 Uterine incision

1. Make a vertical 10 cms incision in the anterior part of the uterus beginning as low as possible, if possible within the lower segment quickly

2. Care should be exercised to avoid cutting the fetus

3. The leg of the fetus is grasped and delivered

4. Estimate blood loss and replace if excessive

3.5 Closing the uterus

1. Close inner myometrial layer

2. Have the assisstant manually approximate the edges

3. Close the mid portion of the myometrium, leaving 1 cm of outer myometrium still open

4. Close the serosa and outer layer using a baseball stitch, which is hemostatic and minimizes exposed raw surfaces, and thus may reduce adhesions

3.6 Techniques to avoid lacerating the fetus

1. Allis clamps to the superior and inferior edges of the myometrial incision and elevate them

2. Directly apply the end of the suction tubing to the center of the myometrial incision to balloon-out and thin-out

3.7 Midline incision fascial closure

1. Use of a simple running technique

2. Use of #1 or #2 delayed absorbable monofilament suture (eg, polydioxanone [PDS])

3. Mass closure of all layers of abdominal wall

4. Wide tissue bites (≥1 cm)

5. Utilization of short tissue interval (≤1 cm)

6. Suture length should be 4 times larger than wound length

7. Use of tension free bites

4. Extracting impacted head

A cesarean section done for later stages labor or prolonged labor, in which the fetal head is impacted in the pelvis, can lead to worse maternal and perinatal outcomes.

4.1 Methods to dis-impact the deeply engaged fetal head include

1. Abdomino-vaginal delivery

2. The reverse breech extraction technique

3. Use of a head elevator

4. Utilization of non-dominant hand for extraction

5. Lowering down the operating table

6. Insertion of a ballon device to disimpact an engaged fetal head before an emergency CD and

7. Patwardhan's shoulders first technique

4.2 General steps

1. Adequate abdominal wall and uterine incisions

2. Adequate uterine relaxation with nitroglycerine

3. Avoiding using fulcrum on the lower uterine segment

4.3 Abdominovaginal delivery (push techniques)

1. Put the mother in Whitmore or Frog position

2. An assistant's hand/dominant hand of the surgeon disimpacts the head

3. The surgeon uses upward traction on the shoulders and avoids fetal head deflection

4. After fetal head is disimpacted delivery through the hysterectomy incision is compeleted

4.4 Reverse breech extraction

If you are taking a mother with prolonged labor for caesarian section, it would be beneficiary if you decide the method to dis-impact the deeply engaged fetal head ahead of time. Thus, localizing the maternal side which the feet of the fetus are located would shorten the precious intraoperative time spent in search of it.

1. Make slightly higher up transverse incision in the uterus

2. Look for the fetal foot

3. Slowly deliver the foot one by one

4. Then deliver the trunk

5. Avoid hyper extension during the delivery of the head of the fetus.

Though there was no statistically significant difference in bladder injury, several systematic reviews and meta-analysis showed that reverse breech extraction is associated with significantly lower maternal risks compared with the push method. Uterine incision extension, infection, mean blood loss, and operative time were significantly higher with the push technique compared with the reverse breech extraction [4, 6–8].

5. Extraction of floating head

Elective cesarean section for fetal growth restriction or for premature fetus may pose difficulty in extraction of the fetal head.

Vacuum or forceps extraction, Coyne spoon assisted delivery, internal podalic version are the techniques for extraction of floating head.

6. Placenta Previa

Placenta previa occurs when the placenta covers the internal uterine orifice. Placenta previa is common risk factor for antepartum and postpartum hemorrhage, postpartum hysterectomies, with increased maternal morbidity and mortality. Cesarean section in the presence of placenta previa is difficult experience. Avoiding placental incision is first rule [9, 10].

Options of management can be:

1. Low vertical avoiding the placenta on one side if placental location is anterolateral

2. J or T shaped uterine incisions for placental shear down

3. Classicial uterine incision

4. Go-through

Lower segment placentation bleeding

1. Figure of-8 sutures in the placental bed
2. Use oxytocine and misoprostol simultaneously
3. Direct injection of Prostaglandin F2

7. Transverse lie

Transverse lie is fetal presentation in which the fetal longitudinal axis lies perpendicular to maternal spine. It affects <1% of pregnancies at term and it is an indication for cesarean section [11–13]. Fetal extraction is the commonest difficulty encountered during the procedure. All women with transverse lie must be admitted at 37 weeks +0 days.

- External cephalic version at 37 weeks +0 days, if successful and recurs a repeat external cephalic version at 38–39 weeks
- If successful at 38–39 weeks
    - Rapture the membrane while the vertex is held in position and start induction
- If no experienced personnel for ECV or the mother refuses
    - Schedule the mother for elective CD at 39–39 weeks +6 days

Dorso-superior (back up) transverse lie

- Skin incision
    - Good free access to the lower uterine segment
- Review fetal lie
    - Try to convert it to longuitidinal
    - Rule out placenta previa
    - Keep the lower uterine segment free of fluids with suction
    - Incise the lower uterine segment
    - Feel for the presenting part
- For the back-up transverse lie in women with a well-developed lower uterine segment
    - Make a low transverse hysterotomy using an accentuated curvilinear incision to reduce the risk of extension into the broad ligament

 - The surgeon standing on the same side as the fetal head then attempts to grasp the fetal feet and perform a footling breech extraction

 - If difficulty is encountered, a vertical incision is made to form an inverted-T

Dorso-inferior (back down) transverse lie

- The dorso-inferior (back down) transverse lie is more difficult to deliver than the back up transverse lie because the fetal feet are difficult to grasp.

- If the fetal membranes are intact,

 - perform an intra-abdominal version to convert the transverse lie to a cephalic or breech presentation before making the hysterotomy, thus facilitating delivery through the low segment accentuated curvilinear transverse uterine incision

 - For the version, one hand is placed on the fetal head and the other hand is placed on the buttocks

 - The fetal pole that will become the presenting part is very gently manipulated toward the pelvic inlet while the other pole is guided in the opposite direction

 - Although either cephalic or podalic version can be performed, we have found that breech extraction is technically easier

 - After the version has been completed, an assistant holds the fetus in the longitudinal position so it will not revert to its original position, the hysterotomy is made, and the fetus is delivered

The assistant performs intraabdominal version prior to hysterotomy and holds the fetus in its new longitudinal position. The surgeon will then perform the lower-segment uterine incision at the dotted line.

After external version from transverse lie to breech, the fetus is extracted in the breech presentation by the operator, while the assistant continuously holds the fetus in longitudinal position.

- Some experts recommend a vertical uterine incision for the back down transverse lie, which is also a reasonable approach. But vertical hysterotomy, even if mostly confined to the lower segment, is less desirable than a transverse incision as it may increase the risk of uterine rupture in a subsequent pregnancy, but it may be necessary if the lower uterine segment is poorly developed [3]

- If the fetus is large, especially if membranes are ruptured and the shoulder is impacted in the birth canal, a classical incision may be necessary

8. Previous CS/surgery with extensive adhesions

Adhesions are common following cesarean delivery and after abdominal surgery. The extent of adhesions varies among individuals. In the presence of adhesions, the cesarean section and fetal extraction are difficult, incision to delivery time is prolonged and the risk of complications such as hemorrhage, bowel or bladder injury is heightened [2, 14, 15].

- Bladder, bowel, and the uterus might be adherent to the sheath
- The most important aspect of adhesions is to try to restore normal anatmoy as far as possible
- Cut and tie of bands
- Cut muscles
- If omentum is adherentt to the peritoneum,
  - Clamp the adhesion, cut and tie it with vicryl
- If the bladder is adherent to uterine wall,
  - Try to open the peritoneal cavity by cutting higher up
- If bowel adhesions are encountered.
  - Try to separate the bowel from the adherent tissue using sharp dissection
- One often has thick fibrous bands extending from the uterus to the rectus muscle
  - Those are also tied and cut through, in order to secure easy access to the lower uterine segment
- In the event of poor exposure to the lower uterine segment cut the bellies of rectus mussle latterally
  - Do not hesitate to call in the help of other specialities and your seniors!
- Perform the hysterotomy in the most appropriate accessible location
- Another option is a paravesical or supravesical extraperitoneal approach

9. Absent lower uterine segment

- This is encountered during
  - Delivery of premature infant
  - Placenta previa

- Classic Incision is preferred
    - Secure hemostasis
    - Close the serosa to avoid adhesions

10. Fibroid uterus

If the fibroid is situated near the lower segment at the uterine incision line it becomes a potential life threatening problem. Will

- In such cases do
    - Vertical lower uterine incision
    - Classical cesarean section

CD in Breech Presentation

- Increase the lower uterine segment exposure
- Introduce your right hand and find the feet
- Perform a gentle breech extraction
- Always keep the baby's back upwards

Author details

Awol Yemane Legesse* and Hale Teka
Department of Obstetrics and Gynecology, College of Health Sciences, Mekelle University, Ethiopia

*Address all correspondence to: hayuawol1@gmail.com

References

[1] Monaghan JM. Bonney's Gynaecological Surgery. 10th ed. Oxford, UK: Blackwell Science Ltd.; 2004

[2] Visconti F, Quaresima P, Rania E, Palumbo AR, Micieli M, Zullo F, et al. Difficult caesarean section: A literature review. European Journal of Obstetrics and Gynecology and Reproductive Biology. 2020;**246**:72-78. DOI: 10.1016/j.ejogrb.2019.12.026

[3] Gary Cunningham F. Williams Obstetrics. 24th ed. NewYork, USA: The McGraw-Hill Companies, Inc; 2012

[4] Jeve YB, Navti OB, Konje JC. Comparison of techniques used to deliver a deeply impacted fetal head at full dilation: A systematic review and meta-analysis. BJOG. 2016;**123**:337-345

[5] Kotsuji F, Knishijima T, Kurokawa Y, Yoshida T, Sekiya M, Banzai H, et al. Transverse uterine fundal incision for placenta previa with accreta, involving the entire anterior uterine wall: Case series. BJOG. 2013;**120**:1144-1149

[6] Levy R, Chernomoretz T, Appelman Z, Levin D, Or Y, Hagay ZJ. Head pushing versus reverse breech extraction in cases of impacted fetal head during cesarean section. Eur J Obstret Gynecol Reprod Biol. 2005;**121**(1):24-26

[7] Fasubaa OB, Ezechi OC, Orji EO, Ogunniyi SO, Akindele ST, Loto OM, et al. Delivery of the impacted head of the fetus at caesarean section after prolonged obstructed labour: A randomised comparative study of two methods. The Obstetrician and Gynaecologist. 2002;**22**(4):375-378

[8] Chopra S, Bagga R, Keepanasseril A, Jain V, Kalra J, Suri V. Disengagement of the deeply engaged fetal head during cesarean section in advanced labor: Conventionl method versus reverse breech extraction. Acta Obstetricia et Gynecologica. 2009;**88**(10):1163-1166

[9] Silver RM. Abnormal placentation: placenta previa, vasa previa, and placenta accreta. Obstetrics and Gynecology. 2015;**126**:654-668

[10] Cunningham FG, Leveno KJ, Bloom SL, et al. Obstetrical hemorrhage. In: Cunningham FG, Leveno KJ, Bloom SL, editors. Williams Obstetrics. 26th ed. New York: McGraw-Hill; 2022. pp. 757-803

[11] Okonofua FE. Management of neglected shoulder presentation. BJOG. 2009;**116**(13):1695-1696

[12] Pilliod RA, Caughey AB. Fetal malpresentation and malposition: Diagnosis and management. Obstetrics and Gynecology Clinics of North America. 2017;**44**:631-643

[13] Shoham Z, Blickstein I, Zosmer A, et al. Transverse uterine incision for cesarean delivery of the transverse-lying fetus. European Journal of Obstetrics, Gynecology, and Reproductive Biology. 1989;**32**:67-70

[14] Silver RM, Landon MB, Rouse DJ, Leveno KJ, Spong CY, Thom EA, et al. Maternal morbidity associated with multiple repeat cesarean deliveries. Obstetrics and Gynecology. 2006;**107**(6):1226-1232

[15] Walfisch A, Beloosesky R, Shrim A, Hallak M. Adhesion prevention after cesarean delivery: Evidence, and lack of it. American Journal of Obstetrics and Gynecology. 2014;**211**(5):446-452

Chapter 6

Complex Cesarean Section

Salvatore Felis, Marta Fiamberti and Chiara Peluffo

Abstract

The cesarean section, in principle, is not a complex surgical procedure when compared to many others performed in our specialty. However, there is a complex set of physiological and anatomical elements and circumstances that must interact perfectly to obtain an optimal result. Surgical technique is a factor but is often not the primary determinant of a positive outcome; concomitant circumstances interact in a cesarean section such as obstructed labor, abruptio placenta, morbid invasion of the placenta, previous pelvic infection, chorioamnionitis/endometritis, chronic and acute anemia, inadequate blood or insufficient transfusion capacity, oxytocics, anesthetics, lack of (or lack of appropriate administration of) antibiotics, and trained or motivated personnel. In all these cases, and in many other contexts, less-than-optimal results may occur, even in the face of a perfect surgical technique.

Keywords: complex cesarean section, adequate resources, inadequate resources, hemorrhage, hysterectomy

1. Introduction

The cesarean section is ideally not a complex surgical procedure compared to many others performed in our specialty. However, a complex set of elements and physiological and anatomical circumstances should/must interact perfectly to obtain a good result. Surgical technique is often not the primary determinant of a positive outcome; the outcome comprehends the interaction of many factors such as obstructed labor, abruptio placenta, placenta previa, previous pelvic infection, chorioamnionitis/endometritis, chronic or acute anemia, insufficient transfusion capacity, oxytocic, anesthetics, absence of antibiotic therapy or wrong choice of antibiotics, and trained or motivated staff. In all these situations and in many other contexts, far from optimal results may occur despite a perfect surgical technique. As the number of cesarean sections in the world is growing, challenging interventions will become the standard rather than the exception. It is mandatory that obstetricians should receive initial and ongoing training focused on recognizing conditions of increased risk and those who are entrusted with the surgery have adequate experience in managing multiple complications frequently associated with a cesarean section. This may involve a revision of the procedures and the development of guidelines appropriate for the referral of cases with the highest risk of complications at these centers of excellence.

2. Cesarean section in environments with adequate resources

2.1 Risks in full dilation cesarean section with absolute dystocia

The risks of a full dilation cesarean section appear to be less important when there is the availability of an operating room and the necessary support services to perform the intervention. While the risks are somehow lowered in this scenario, all the associated complications should be anticipated. A large retrospective cohort study conducted in Nova Scotia [1] assessed 55,273 births, comprising 549 full dilation cesarean sections. Authors proved that women who underwent a full dilation C-section were more likely to experience intraoperative trauma and perinatal asphyxiation compared to the ones who underwent a cesarean section during the first stage of labor (OR, 2.57; 95% CI, 1.71–3.88 and OR, 1.5; 95% CI, 1.06–2.14). These results confirm that, even in high-level hospital settings, maternal and neonatal outcomes can be adversely affected by prolonged labor, leading to a full dilation cesarean section. Another study involved 627 singleton pregnancies in nulliparous women who underwent an emergency cesarean section in the UK; of these, 199 (18.9%) had a full dilatation cesarean section [2]. Intraoperative complications and blood transfusions were more likely to occur in women undergoing a full dilation cesarean section (OR, 4.6; 95% CI, 2.7–7.9 and OR, 2.9; 95% CI, 1.5–5.6). Apart from that, there were no differences in terms of the incidence of new hospitalization, hospitalization longer than 5 days, or perinatal morbidity between the two groups. Another small retrospective study conducted at Singapore on 110 emergency full dilation cesarean sections showed no statistically significant adverse maternal or fetal outcomes [3]. It is not uncommon for the bladder to be injured or lacerated during a cesarean section for protracted or obstructed labor. Once the lesion is recognized, the bladder can be fixed with a two-layer closure; if the ureters or the bladder trine is damaged, urological consultation has to be performed, and if it is not available, the patient should be immediately transferred to a center where it can be done. After the repair of the bladder injury, a urinary catheter should be left in for at least 7–10 days.

2.2 Rupture of the uterus

Rupture of the uterus during labor has dramatic consequences for both the mother and the fetus; following the uterine rupture, the fetus passes into the abdominal cavity with low chances of survival unless rapid intervention is performed. This situation is often accompanied by some degree of placental abruption. If the patient is admitted to a high-level hospital, early identification of the rupture—one of the first signs is abnormal fetal heart rate on CTG [4]—and delivery within 18 minutes [5] by laparotomy can prevent fetal death and the onset of neurological complications. Risks of hypoxic ischemic encephalopathy and perinatal death with uterus rupture stand at 6.8% (1.8–10.6%) and 1.8% (0.0-4%,2%), respectively [6, 7]. Women who decide to undergo a TOLAC (trial of labor after cesarean) should be informed about the risk of uterine rupture during labor; for women with a previous Pfannenstiel incision, this risk is about 1% and increases between 4 and 9% for those with a classic scar [8]. Uterine rupture rarely occurs in women who have never undergone full-thickness uterine surgery, especially in a low-resource environment, after prolonged obstructed labor and increased uterine contractions [9].

2.3 Pathological obesity

Obesity is a risk factor for a cesarean section. Considering the obesity epidemic, it is not surprising that doctors are increasingly called upon to perform cesarean sections for obese women (BMI ≥ 30) [10, 11]. The results of a secondary analysis of the FASTER study indicate that a cesarean section is more common in obese and morbidly obese individuals than in normal weight subjects (20.7 vs. 33.8 vs. 47.4%, respectively) [12]. A cesarean section in morbidly obese subjects involves an increased risk of complications such as increased technical difficulty of the surgical procedure, poor wound healing, and increased potential risk of venous thromboembolism [13]. The need for a cesarean section is due to both maternal and fetal factors: the greater difficulty in monitoring fetal heart rate and a more likely dystocia of labor lead to the execution of an earlier and more complex cesarean section. During surgery, the surgeon must assess the skin incision, balancing the most efficient extraction of the fetus and optimal wound healing (**Figure 1**).

Rather than a vertical midline incision, the Pfannenstiel or Joel-Cohen incision is associated with less abdominal tension and less complications in situations of increased intra-abdominal pressure, such as a chronic cough. In a morbidly obese woman with a large abdominal panniculus, wound healing may be impaired due to the continued presence of moisture in the area. If the adipose panniculus is not mobile or the anatomy of the abdomen is altered, it should be better to make a supra-umbilical incision, over the anterior and fundic portion of the uterus, in order to facilitate fetal extraction. This approach has to be preferred in women who opt for tubal ligation and who do not plan further pregnancies as high uterine incisions are associated with a greater risk of subsequent uterus ruptures. Regardless of the type of incision, the current recommendations provide for the execution of a subcutaneous suture when the subcutaneous fat has a thickness greater than 2 cm, to prevent the formation of a seroma and the dehiscence of the wound. If the incision is subjected to a large amount of moisture due to the presence of skin folds, it is wise to leave a dressing covering the healing skin until the risk of wound. Dehiscence has reduced, to avoid the formation of a seroma [14]. In contrast, there is no evidence that subcutaneous drainage is effective in preventing postoperative morbidity.

Additional considerations must be taken into account when performing a cesarean section on morbidly obese individuals. A pragmatically important indication is to

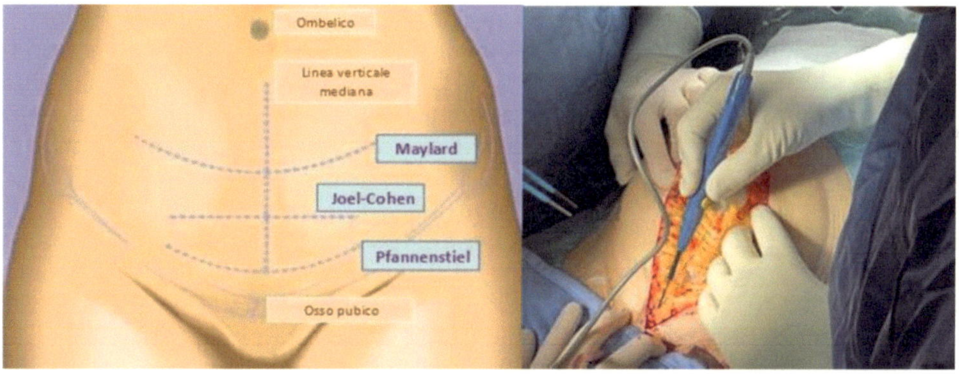

Figure 1.
Laparotomic abdominal incisions. a. (left) Representation of variants. b. (right) Xifopubic incision.

make sure that the operating table can support the patient's weight, especially when tilted or placed in the Trendelenburg position. While lying in a supine position, a patient may experience shortness of breath. This sensation may not be relieved by releasing the pressure of the uterus on the inferior vena cava with the insertion of a wedge to maintain the left lateral tilt position. In these situations, raising the head of the bed by 15°–20° is sufficient to relieve the feeling of shortness of breath. Obesity affects anesthesia choices; it may not be possible to apply epidural analgesia due to inadequate length of the spinal needle, inability to reach anatomical landmarks, and irregular distribution of drugs in the blood. If regional anesthesia is ineffective or impossible, the patient must undergo general anesthesia, which involves its own risks, including aspiration of gastric material and transplacental transfer of drugs. Since there is an increased risk of venous thromboembolism, both mechanical and pharmacological prophylaxis must be performed in morbidly obese women. Finally, due attention should be paid to the administration of correct antibiotic dosage, taking into account the potentially increased volume of distribution of these drugs.

2.4 Uterine leiomyomas

The incidence of uterine leiomyomas in pregnancy ranges from 0.1 to 3.9% [15, 16]. Uterine leiomyomas can cause various complications during pregnancy, including recurrent miscarriage, preterm birth, premature birth, premature rupture of membranes (PROM), and malpresentation. Furthermore, large uterine myomas are at risk of degeneration during pregnancy, leading to inflammation and pain accompanying the degenerative process. Furthermore, women with uterine leiomyomas were more likely to experience complications of labor and delivery, such as dysfunctional or prolonged labor, breech presentation, and cesarean delivery (OR, 1.90; 95% CI, 1.65–2.18); women with leiomyomas were more likely to require a cesarean section than women whose uterus was of regular morphology (OR, 7.59; 95% CI, 5.47–10.53). Even with medical indications for a cesarean section, women with uterine leiomyomas were much more likely to require a cesarean section (OR, 5.26; 95% CI, 3.98–6.95). A systematic review examining the influence of uterine leiomyomas on the whole course of pregnancy showed that the difficulties of a cesarean section depend on the number and location of the fibroids [16]. In a study based on hospital records among women who gave birth between 1987 and 1993 in Washington (USA), the prevalence of diagnosed uterine leiomyoma was 0.37% [15]. The study showed that women with uterine leiomyomas were more likely to have pregnancy complications, including first-trimester bleeding, placental abruption, and PROM (OR, 1.87; 95% CI, 1.59–2.20). Several factors must be taken into consideration when determining the best way to deliver: women with single pregnancy and a single large fibroid should undergo a primary cesarean section if the fetal head is unable to pass the myoma and engage in the pelvis. If the uterine myoma involves a significant portion of the lower uterine segment, thus making a low transverse incision difficult or impossible to access through the uterus, the only viable and safe option may be a classic incision. The safety of myomectomy at the time of a cesarean section has long been debated due to the possibility of uncontrollable bleeding following the removal of uterine myomas in the presence of increased vascularity during pregnancy [17]. A retrospective case–control study of 120 women with uterine leiomyomas present during delivery included 40 women who underwent myomectomy at the time of a cesarean section and 80 controls without myomectomy [16]. The authors defined an excessive intraoperative blood loss as both a drop in hematocrit of 10 points or more from the preoperative value and the need for a transfusion. The surgical technique was described as follows: "A linear incision was made on the myoma and electrocautery was used to remove the myomas with minimal blood loss. The closure of the myometrium was made in one or two layers using absorbable broken sutures (1/0 vicryl caliber). The serosa is sutured using a continuous absorbable suture (2/0 or 3/0 vicryl caliber)." Women who had undergone myomectomy at the time of cesarean section had statistically larger uterine leiomyomas compared to those who did not have a myomectomy (8.1 ± 4.7 cm vs. 5.7 ± 2.7 cm, $P < 0.05$). There was no statistically significant difference in the rate of bleeding (12.5% vs. 11.3%) or postoperative fever (defined as temperature ≥ 38.0° C; 7.5% vs. 10%), while myomectomy involved longer operations (53.3 ± 18.6 minutes vs. 44, 4 ± 6.7 minutes, $P < 0.05$) and a longer length of hospitalization (3.3 ± 0.8 gi hours vs. 2.7 ± 0.6 days, $P < 0.05$). A large university hospital in China has adopted the policy of routine myomectomy at the time of a cesarean section for women with uterine leiomyomas; a retrospective study was subsequently performed to evaluate the safety and efficacy of the procedure [18]. A total of 1967 pregnant women also had uterine fibroids, 1438 of whom underwent a cesarean section (73.1%): 1242 (86.4%) were simultaneously subjected to myomectomy, 51 (5.3%) to hysterectomy, and 145 (10.1%) underwent only a cesarean section. The surgical technique has been described extensively, and electrocautery has not been used. Excessive bleeding was defined as a 10% decrease in hematocrit or the need for intraoperative transfusion. Women who had a cesarean section associated with hysterectomy had leiomyomas of a larger mean diameter (8.1 ± 3.9 cm) than women who underwent myomectomy at the time of a cesarean section (7.3 ± 4.6 cm) and women undergoing a cesarean section without myomectomy (3.6 ± 2.1 cm). There were no significant differences between the three groups in terms of length of hospitalization. The mean length of hospitalization, even routine, among patients with a cesarean section without myomas was quite long (4.9 ± 1.9 days). There were also no significant differences between the groups in the frequency of bleeding or the incidence of post-operative fever (defined as temperature ≥ 38.0°C). The duration of surgery was longer in women undergoing myomectomy at the time of a cesarean section (83.6 ± 10.8 minutes) compared to a cesarean section in women without uterine leiomyomas (40.2 ± 8.9 minutes) and a cesarean section in women with uterine leiomyomas (41.9 ± 9.1 minutes). Cumulative data suggest that, in appropriately selected pregnant women, myomectomy can be performed safely at the time of a cesarean section without concern for uncontrolled bleeding or post-operative fever. However, the optimal technique to use in the context of a cesarean section remains unclear, as several techniques are described, including the use of tourniquets and electrocautery. Patients should be informed of the longer operating time and length of hospital stay when a myomectomy is performed.

2.5 Pelvic adhesive disease

The formation of an adhesion is a complex process that results from the imbalance between the deposition of fibrin and its disintegration during the healing process. Most of the adhesions rise during the first postoperative week. While opening the abdomen, the obstetrician could sometimes be faced with severe pelvic adhesions, which can be the result of previous cesarean sections, pelvic inflammatory disease, or bowel, bladder, and gynecological surgeries. Unless there is an immediate danger to the fetal condition, it would be better to restore the anatomy before performing the cesarean section even if there could be a greater risk of sectioning the underlying bowel or bladder. When faced with impenetrable adhesions, it is advisable to make a higher incision in order to expose non-scarred tissue; once the abdomen has been entered and the distinct structures recognized, an orderly approach can be undertaken. The option of an inverted T incision, a J incision, or even a separate supraumbilical incision should be taken under consideration. If adhesions make the lower uterine segment completely inaccessible, a fundus or even a posterior uterine incision may be required to deliver the newborn. The presence of adhesions during the cesarean section increases with each subsequent operation and affects both the time of delivery of the newborn and the overall surgical operating time. A recent study showed that in the presence of adhesions, the delivery time was increased by 18.2, 20.3, and 27.5 minutes, respectively, from the second to the fourth delivery [19]. When the abdomen is full of severe, extensive, and dense adhesions, delivery times increase by 8.4, 12.6, and 21.5 minutes from the second to the fourth cesarean section compared to the first cesarean section. The proportional decrease in the pH values of the umbilical cord and in Apgar scores was reported in newborns delivered after a woman already underwent multiple cesarean sections. This study was limited by its retrospective nature and reliance on the interpretation of surgical reports, but the presence and severity of adhesion suggest a potential impact on fetal well-being as a consequence of cesarean sections. These results are consistent with another retrospective review showing that delivery times are significantly increased by 3–5 minutes as the number of cesarean sections increases [20]. The surgical technique focused on the prevention of postoperative adhesions has been studied with variable results, including the closure or non-closure of the rectus muscles and the peritoneum. The presence of intraperitoneal and bladder adhesions has been related to the creation of a bladder flap at the time of hysterotomy; in conclusion, the creation of a bladder flap causes inflammation and fibrotic reaction, that leads to the activation of reactive processes and the release of regenerative mesothelial agent with a subsequent subomesothelial hyperplasia and fibrosis [21]. The same authors, as well as others, have suggested that the closure of the visceral peritoneum during a cesarean section can produce an inflammatory reaction and adhesions [22, 23]. Therefore, scientific evidence seems to support the non-creation of a bladder flap and the non-closure of the visceral peritoneum at the time of hysterectomy and uterine closure. A recent study has suggested that the presence of severe striae gravidarum may indicate the presence of underlying intraperitoneal adhesions in women who have had a previous cesarean section [24]. The authors used the Davey striae gravidarum score to quantify the severity of the striae and found that 50% of women with severe striae and a previous cesarean section had intraperitoneal adhesions versus 9% of women without striae. Similarly, the relationship between keloid presence and adhesion formation among women of different races was examined [20]: while adhesion formation appears to be comparable, women with cesarean scar keloids have more adhesions between the uterus and the anterior abdominal wall.

2.6 Abnormal fetal station/fetus not engaged

Understanding the fetal station, presentation, and position of the head prior to entry into the abdomen or uterus saves valuable minutes at delivery by enabling a strategic approach to surgery. Advantages include proper planning of the incision and correct positioning of the hand, which allow for the best grasp and flexion of the fetal head in the case of cephalic birth (or of the feet in the case of breech birth) and to ensure that any additional maneuvers, such as forceps or suction cups, are available in the room for quick use.

2.7 Fetal head not engaged

When an uncommitted or "floating" fetal head is encountered, it can be difficult to guide the head to a transverse uterine incision, in particular when the fetal head deflects. In this case, the use of a suction cup or forceps can be particularly useful in extracting the fetus. However, it is not always possible to know when the forceps or the suction cup will be needed, and if these instruments are not part of the normal cesarean section set, it is advisable to have them available in the operating room to avoid a delayed extraction caused by the recovery of these instruments. To apply a suction cup at the time of a cesarean section, the same general principles should be followed as for operative vaginal delivery. Almost all types of forceps can be used at the time of a cesarean section; however, long handles and standard handles can create problems in its use, and it is therefore advisable to use forceps with short handles and handles during a cesarean delivery. The technique for applying these tools is different from the one used in the vagina. First, the fetal head must be palpated to determine presentation; once the presentation is confirmed, the posterior blade should be guided under the fetal head and held in place by the assistant. Only at this time can the anterior blade be positioned: depending on the maternal anatomy and the type of forceps available, the anterior blade can be placed directly on the fetal head, or it may be necessary to position it posteriorly and guide it into position before locking the handles. It is important to lock the handles before exerting any traction on the blades. Finally, the surgical assistant should provide pressure on the fundus of the uterus while gentle upward traction of the forceps is exerted, guiding the fetus out of the hysterotomy; conversely, pulling down and toward the mother's feet can cause an extension of the hysterotomy.

2.8 Transverse posterior spine situation

Delivery of a fetus in a transverse posterior position is technically challenging and often requires a classic incision. When transverse uterine incisions are attempted for this presentation, it is often necessary to use a J incision or a T incision on the uterus to extract the infant. Extension of the uterine incision is associated with increased blood loss, broad ligament hematoma, and uterine artery tear [25]; thus, the preoperative execution of an ultrasound for the evaluation of the fetus, when the presentation is uncertain, can be the key to a safe birth.

2.9 Perimortem cesarean section

The incidence of cardiac arrest in pregnancy in the United States from 1998 to 2011 was estimated to be 1 in 12,000 pregnant women [26], and although this number is quite low, it is higher than the most recent estimated incidence in the United Kingdom of 1:20,000 [27]. This increase is potentially attributable to a number of causes, including an increase in pregnant women with acquired or congenital heart disease, who survive to a reproductive age, and events such as acute bleeding, amniotic fluid embolism, and sepsis. An international consensus on cardiopulmonary resuscitation and cardiovascular emergency care, in 2010, established therapeutic recommendations trying to determine if any specific interventions would improve the outcome of pregnant women in cardiac arrest [28]. During full-term pregnancy, occlusion of the inferior vena cava by the uterus and fetus is significant, resulting in a 30% decrease in blood volume for the pregnant woman compared to that of a non-pregnant woman [28]. Placing pregnant women on a left lateral inclined plane, to prevent aorto-caval compression by the pregnant uterus, has numerous maternal and fetal benefits in non-arrest situations:

- For the mother: increased blood pressure and cardiac output.
- For the fetus: better oxygenation and a non-stress situation.

The sum of these benefits suggests that positioning on a left lateral inclined plane should be desirable in the case of cardiac arrest to improve maternal and fetal status during resuscitation; however, the method chosen to position the woman in a left lateral tilt during chest compressions may be important for maternal survival. There are few clinical studies on resuscitation techniques for pregnant women. In a systematic review [27], only two studies were identified that used manikins to test the effectiveness of chest compression. These studies suggest that although chest compressions can be performed in the left lateral inclination position, they are not as effective as those performed in the supine position: with the increase in the inclination angle, the effectiveness of chest compressions decreases. Considering the importance of effective and uninterrupted chest compressions in maintaining the perfusion of critical organs, the authors recommend manual displacement of the uterus as a valid alternative to the left lateral tilt position, stressing that the former is equally effective in relieving caval compression during cesarean delivery in patients not in arrest [27]. For the mother, the extraction of the fetus and the afterbirth of the placenta can lead to a rapid improvement in the hemodynamic state, including the return of the pulse and the improvement of blood pressure. Maternal resuscitation is in fact improved from delivery, allowing more blood to return to the heart through the inferior vena cava once the fetus has been extracted [28]. Immediate extraction is even more important when you have a viable fetus, as quick action can make a difference in its survival. Based on data collected between 1900 and 1985, delivery of a viable fetus within 5 minutes of the mother's cardiac arrest is associated with survival with intact neurological status [29], while newborns delivered more than 5 minutes after the onset of arrest are more likely to undergo neurological sequelae, the severity of which appears less with increasing gestational age. A perimortem cesarean section should be performed normally but with an emergency character [29]: time should not be wasted in determining fetal heart tones, since the extraction of the fetus from the uterus guarantees greater chances of fetal and maternal survival. The patient may or may not be moved to the operating room, depending on the logistics and time required for transit; since the procedure will be essentially bloodless, due to the absence of maternal cardiac output, the surgery can be performed in almost all places with relative ease. Only after the extraction of the fetus, with the return of cardiac output, and the consequent appearance of blood loss, the closure of the various abdominal layers must comply, as efficiently as possible, with the standard procedure. In general, a vertical skin incision is recommended because of the speed with which the fetus can be extracted, but ultimately, any type of incision that can be done quickly should be done. Where defibrillation is required, the absence of difference in transthoracic impedance during pregnancy suggests that the standard adult energy settings appear appropriate [26], although the study making such observations was performed on an undersized patient sample [27].

2.10 Management of morbidly adherent placenta

Morbid attachment of the placenta (MAP) can encompass many forms ranging from small focal areas of attachment, which may not be recognized, to overt trophoblastic invasion of the bladder or other structures. Some complications can occur in both these situations. Difficult removal of a placenta at the time of a cesarean section should always suggest an MAP; in such cases, it is necessary to prepare what is necessary to stop a possible bleeding (which can develop before, during, and after the closure of the hysterotomy), to perform a blood transfusion, and to prevent the development of coagulopathy. Even small focal areas of placenta accreta can weaken uterine integrity and predispose to placental bed rupture, broad ligament hemorrhage, and development of intramyometrial hematoma. In the recognition of a focal MAP, observation of the placental bed and an in-depth evaluation of the uterine wall are fundamental; in most cases, the use of hemostatic sutures will be sufficient to control bleeding but if these fail, O'Leary-type uterine artery ligation [30], uterine compression sutures (B-Lynch or some modification thereof), or gradual devascularization [31]. Ongoing bleeding, despite these efforts, should lead to a necessary reassessment of the strategy. In the presence of dangerous bleeding and a persistent risk to maternal life, a hysterectomy must be performed as a last resort, and appropriate measures must be taken for this type of surgery. In such cases, arterial embolization is not an option, given the temporal latency of this procedure and the consequent risk of delays. Very important is the development of algorithms for the treatment of postpartum hemorrhage and the establishment of regular training and simulation courses to ensure staff readiness and familiarity with the disease. Once a decision has been made for an emergency hysterectomy, sustained pressure on the bleeding areas can allow the bleeding to be contained sufficiently to ensure resuscitation and preparation for the procedure. In cases where rapid and safe surgical access to the uterine and utero-ovarian arteries is possible, early clamping or ligation of these vessels (via O'Leary-type sutures or progressively higher lateral uterine sutures) can reduce the loss of blood. In any case, as long as preparations for definitive surgery are in place, blood loss should be attenuated in order to stabilize the patient, maintaining a good hemodynamic situation and normal coagulation and electrolyte parameters [32]. The intervention performed more often is as follows: direct uterine compression – B-Lynch suture [31] – direct aortic compression – endo-aortic balloon placement [33] – crossed aortic clamping. In those situations in which the bleeding continues persistently, the hemorrhage of the placental bed can be controlled with the implementation of hemostatic sutures and, after the hysterotomy has been closed, with the inflation of a Bakri-type balloon. Following inflation of the balloon with sterile saline, the hysterotomy suture can be visually inspected and its integrity checked. Particular attention should be paid to progressive distension of the lower uterine segment (including after contraction of the upper segment or balloon placement), as such distension suggests that there is ongoing bleeding and may signal the need for further procedures. In those hospital units where arterial embolization instruments are available in the operating room and in the presence of a hemodynamically stable patient, the use of selective arterial embolization is very effective in controlling bleeding. In those contexts where this procedure is not feasible, it is recommended to proceed with the hysterectomy rather than transporting the patient to a radiology department where rapid hysterectomy cannot be performed. Sometimes, focal MAP is recognized only once most of the placenta has been removed, with areas of deep invasion found; when accompanied by massive bleeding, this circumstance becomes one of the most dangerous situations in obstetrics. In these cases, there is a rapid deterioration of vital parameters and hemodynamic instability; therefore, the workload of both the surgical and anesthetic teams increases exponentially, often with delays in communicating the mutual needs. Concerted efforts for effective interteam communication will ensure that both teams have minute-by-minute situational awareness and the ability to coordinate their actions. Rapid recognition of the need for hysterectomy is essential, and all efforts should be directed to performing this procedure with minimal blood loss; in the immediate future, blood loss can be minimized by applying pressure to the infrared portion of the aorta and with bimanual uterine compression. If these efforts succeed in reducing bleeding, they could allow the patient to be resuscitated and stabilized so that definitive surgery can be performed. The start of a massive transfusion protocol should be practiced in all units where a C-section is performed; both before and after the infusion of red blood cells, it is necessary to measure and determine the basal electrolyte levels (in particular potassium and calcium), blood count, and coagulation profile. If conservative management fails, the team has to proceed with the hysterectomy, and a post-operative investigation should be performed for any surgical complications (section or ureter ligature, bladder or intestinal injury, nerve injury or development of bruising). The general principles regarding emergency surgery for placenta accreta include those described below. The following suggestions are in most cases anecdotal, gathered from about 50 years of operational experience and from the results of the international literature [30–35].

2.10.1 Surgical preparation for prenatal assessment of MAP

- The pregnant woman must be hospitalized between 33 and 34 weeks of gestation with a planned C-section between 34 and 35 weeks and subsequent hysterectomy.

- Preoperative consultation and planning for surgery and subsequent care should be performed by a multidisciplinary team that includes a midwife, a gynecologist surgeon, an anesthetist, a urologist, an interventional radiologist, a neonatologist, an ICU specialist, and a hematologist. It is important to have a designated team and standard operating procedures to handle patients even in emergency settings.

- It is essential to establish the degree of postpartum hemorrhage, have adequate massive transfusion protocols, and have frequent simulations to keep the team well trained.

- It is necessary to place an arterial line, which will be used to monitor blood pressure, to collect specimen and to place a central venous catheter.

- If possible, ureteral stents should be placed bilaterally to help intraoperative identification of the ureters, which are frequently displaced or deviated by the protruding lower uterine segment.

- Patients should be placed in a lithotomic position with low stirrups to allow visualization of vaginal bleeding and, if necessary, to allow a third co-surgeon to access the surgical field.

- The abdominal access should consist of a peri-umbilical abdominal incision in the midline, with delicate exteriorization of the pregnant uterus to allow classical posterior or fundic hysterotomy.

- No attempt to remove the placenta should be made when there is a suspicion of MAP.

- In those situations where a high-level facility is not available nearby, the C-section should be performed through an incision as far from the placenta as possible. No attempt to remove the placenta should be made, and the uterus should be closed with the placenta in place.

- In those cases where the placental site is not bleeding and the patient is stable, this approach is safer than proceeding with the hysterectomy in an unprepared setting. If the placenta remains in place, the patient must remain in the hospital for at least the first few weeks of observation to avoid postpartum hemorrhage and sepsis.

- There are reports of resection of the placenta and part of the myometrium and reconstitution of the uterus in patients in whom the placenta is not praevia and it is possible to isolate the MAP region [34].

- If the patient starts bleeding during the C-section and hysterectomy (or resection) appears to be necessary, as a life-saving intervention, every effort should be focused on reducing bleeding as much as possible. Methods such as intermittent aorta compression, crossed blockage of aorta, the placement of an aortic balloon catheter, and uterine and pelvic compression should be utilized, until blood transfusion or further help is not available.

2.10.2 MAP surgical technique

- One of the most important aspects of C-section in the case of suspected or known placenta accreta is refraining from trying to remove it. Since a greater risk of MAP is increasingly recognized in women undergoing uterine surgery, performing a second trimester ultrasound can allow early detection of this condition and adequate preparation for childbirth. In conclusion, discovering an MAP at the time of delivery should become a less common occurrence.

- Common practices such as delayed umbilical cord clamping and spontaneous placental abruption at the time of a C-section can actually have an unintended positive effect. Waiting longer before attempting manual placental removal allows the clinician to monitor spontaneous placental separation and closely observe the uterus. In the case of a placenta that does not separate at the time of a C-section, after an appropriate waiting time, the clinician should hypothesize an MAP. This approach can be taught and will become the norm over time; a number of evidence support this strategy. A partial separation of the placenta with a partial removal of the placenta in a fragmented way and the creation of a forced separation plane in the myometrium switch a stable and reasonable situation to an emerging and life-threatening scenario for the woman with fewer options available.

- Similarly, if areas of thinned myometrium or dilated venous sinuses are observed on the surface of the uterus, even in a patient who does not have a history of multiple uterine surgeries, the best approach is not to apply excessive traction to the cord or attempt to remove a placenta that is not separating spontaneously.

- Reproductive technologies have recently been found to significantly increase the risk of MAP; this observation may explain the increase in the incidence of MAP in women at their first birth.

- Due to the abnormal anatomy observed in MAP, the technique of a C-section and hysterectomy is very different from that for an atonic uterus. Due to the very thin lining of the myometrium covering a highly vascularized placental tissue, placing clamps close to the sides of the uterus may result in tearing of the vascular peduncle and underlying uterine tissue, with the exposure of the placental mass and a consequent massive hemorrhage. For this reason, in the case of severe placenta accreta, it is essential to perform a wider lateral pelvic dissection of the broad ligament: the round ligaments and the utero-ovarian are ligated, if possible, after closing the uterus. Whether other myometrial regions are invaded, it is required to separate them from the surrounding tissue. After this step, which reduces blood flow to the uterus, most of the blood from the uterus goes through the uterine arteries, upper bladder arteries, cervicovaginal arteries, and vessels developed through the collateral circulation due to the placenta.

- Before performing hysterectomy in a patient with percreta placenta and clear lateral invasion, or in cases with significant myometrial swelling (indicating a myometrium almost completely replaced by placental tissue), it is recommended to open the retroperitoneal spaces, lateral and parallel to the round ligaments. This step allows an adequate border of avascular parametria to be left between the thinned uterine wall and the vascular peduncle and allows for the safe identification of ureters and retroperitoneal structures. Before ligating the uterine arteries, ureterolysis is performed, and an attempt is made to ligate the artery lateral to the ureter; it may be helpful to use a bipolar cauterizer.

- It is advisable to administer blood products early at the first sign of severe bleeding according to a massive transfusion protocol (transfusion of red blood cells and fresh frozen plasma in a 1:2 ratio). When transfusion is performed, it is important that electrolyte levels are measured frequently, especially calcium and potassium; in the case of placenta percreta, every 20–30 minutes, the following must be performed: arterial blood gas analysis, potassium, calcium, magnesium, complete blood count, prothrombin time and partial thromboplastin time, fibrinogen, D-dimer, and glucose. The platelet count should ideally be above 100,000/mL.

- The placement of intra-abdominal drainages to reveal any further bleeding is not usually necessary but can be useful in the case of doubts.

2.11 Specific considerations in placenta percreta

- It is important to be aware that the blood supply to the lower uterine segment is extremely abnormal in the case of a placenta percreta. Frequently, the same bladder tissue supplies arterial blood to the placenta and drains venous blood through a network of tiny vessels that individually appear insignificant. However, the totality of the surface of these vessels exceeds that of the uterine artery itself. The interface between the bladder tissue and the uterus involved in a placenta percreta must be treated with the same caution as a pulsating artery or a distended vein. Usually, these new vessels have a thin muscular layer, and trying to cauterize them with a diathermocoagulator can cause problems. It is also contraindicated to perform a blunt dissection of the invasion areas because this maneuver can cause massive bleeding (**Figures 2** and **3**).

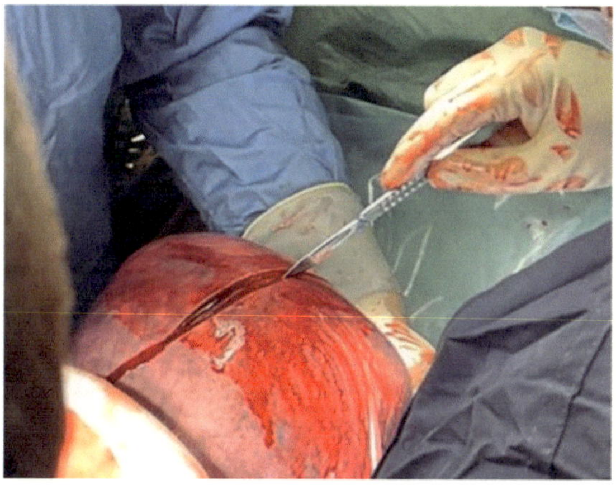

Figure 2.
Fundic incision in the face of a low placental insertion.

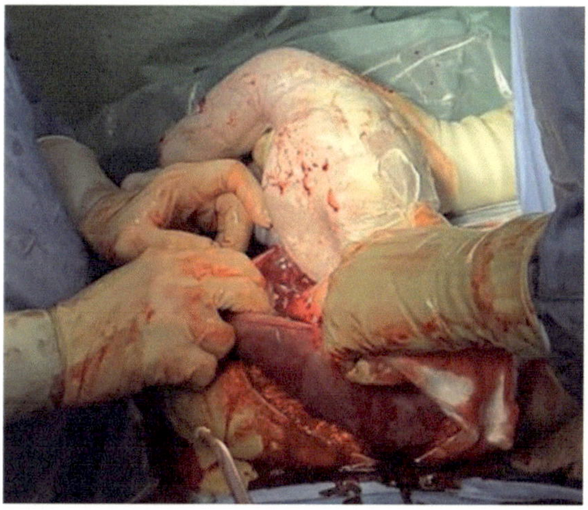

Figure 3.
Subsequent breech extraction of the fetus.

- Whenever possible, a careful and thorough dissection of the bladder tissue from the myometrium with a bipolar cautery device (LigaSure) is preferable in order to retain as much bladder wall as possible. The device allows to clamp small pieces of vascular tissue, to dry the tissue mass, and to separate the two interface zones. Using this technique, it is often necessary to support and suture the bladder wall after completing the hysterectomy due to significant bladder thinning and damage; sometimes, a cystotomy and excision of the attached piece of bladder are done. This approach is preferable to persistent bladder dissection attempts in cases of deep placental invasion (**Figure 4**).

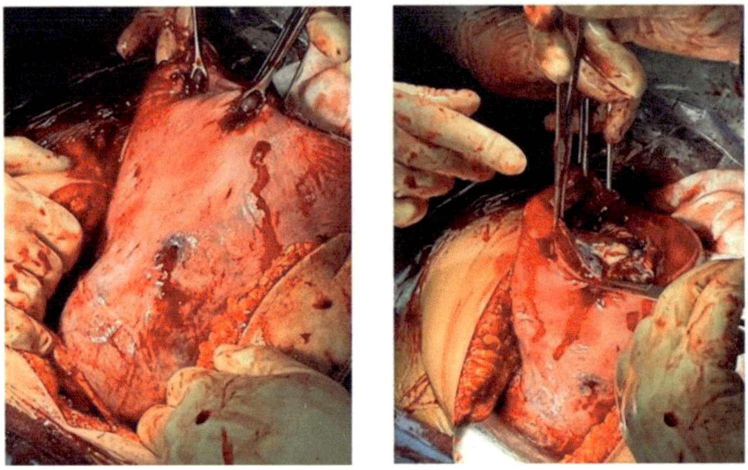

Figure 4.
Placenta firmly adhering to the anterior aspect of the lower uterine segment (left) left in situ (right).

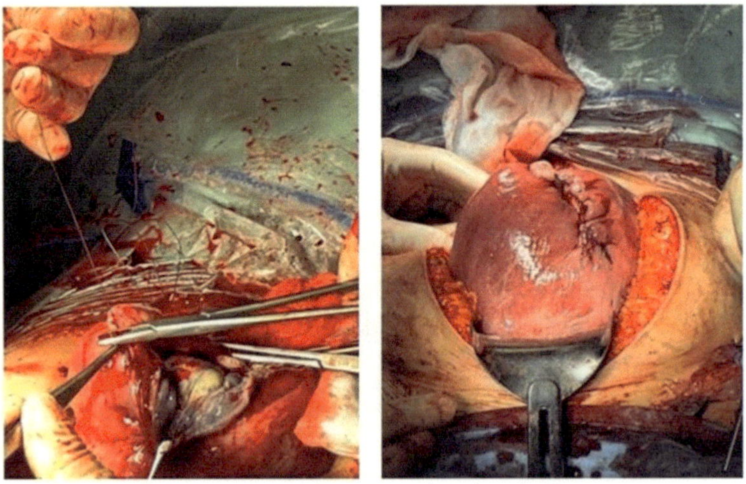

Figure 5.
Fundus closure with placenta left in situ (left). Completion of the fundus suture (right).

- Intraoperative arterial embolization of the placental bed (after a C-section but before hysterectomy) may be necessary when the placenta percreta involves the lateral pelvic walls and dissection seems too risky (**Figure 5**).

Figures of surgical steps.

2.12 Post-surgical assistance

- In those facilities that have an intensive care unit, it is preferable to admit these patients after surgery. Frequently, a massive transfusion is performed, and electrolyte imbalances are present that require correction and minimal monitoring.

- Secondary bleeding is always a possibility in the first hours after surgery; therefore, close monitoring of vital parameters (blood pressure, heart rate, and diuresis) is essential.

- In the case of long-lasting surgery with massive fluid loss and fluid redistribution, prolonged postoperative intubation and assisted ventilation are advisable to reduce the risk of pulmonary edema and respiratory difficulties.

- If minimal residual bleeding is suspected, causing a small collection of intra-abdominal blood, it is recommended to use blood and blood products to resuscitate the patient and correct any coagulopathy. Infusion of large volumes of crystalloids in such patients will produce an expansion of the intravascular volume, a temporary increase in blood pressure, and a decrease in heart rate. This situation is usually temporary, and it will be necessary to bring the patient back to the operating room, because crystalloid infusion causes hemodilution and the reduction of the intravascular concentration of coagulation factors with consequent collection of blood clots in the abdomen, leading to abdominal distension and worsening of the hemoperitoneum. Patients often need to be reoperated only for the hemoperitoneum to be drained. The source of bleeding is usually not detected, and the patient can be closed without further problems once the hemoperitoneum is drained.

2.13 Retroperitoneal hemorrhage during a cesarean section

The most common cause of retroperitoneal hemorrhage at the time of a C-section is the extension of a hysterotomy in the broad ligament with injury to the uterine artery. This lesion may be unrecognized for some time, and often, it is discovered once the blood loss is significant and may have caused the formation of hematomas. In most cases, unless there is an immediate need to drain the blood collection into the retroperitoneum, the safest and most effective way to control bleeding may be the embolization of the uterine arteries or other supply arteries. Attempting to locate the bleeding vessel within an established retroperitoneal hematoma is difficult; if possible and only if the patient is hemodynamically stable, selective embolization may be an option. If embolization is ineffective or impractical and in the presence of continuous life-threatening bleeding, it may become impossible to avoid surgery. In this case, regardless of the initial incision, it is preferable to make a midline abdominal incision, to allow access to the upper retroperitoneum; it is necessary to include in the team a vascular surgeon who can resort to methods such as aortic compression, aortic cross-locking, and the positioning of intraortic balloon devices [32, 33]. It is preferable to enter the retroperitoneum at the top and where there is no hematoma in order to correctly identify the vascular structures and the possible source of the bleeding. In an unstable patient with coagulopathy, compression of the pelvic structures to temporarily reduce blood loss may provide time for life-saving resuscitation. The placement of a pelvic pressure gauze pack [35] or a balloon device to compress the pelvic lateral walls [36] may allow additional time for the aforementioned resuscitation efforts. The combination of pelvic pressure and embolization can allow definitive control of the bleeding.

3. C-section in low-resource countries

Most of the complications seen in well-resourced obstetric settings also occur in limited-resource settings, often with a higher incidence. Fetal heart rate monitoring during labor is relatively rare in contexts with limited resources, as it is infrequent to perform a C-section due to impaired fetal conditions; most urgent or emergent cesarean sections are performed for obstructed labor, antepartum hemorrhage, and uterine rupture. Prolonged labor is followed by dehydration, anemia, infection, and sepsis. The uterus is often edematous and ischemic, with areas of bleeding in the myometrium, and in many of these cases, fetal death has already occurred. Stabilization of the maternal condition prior to surgery is crucial in patients with precarious balance. An urgent C-section performed to attempt to rescue a compromised fetus must be carefully weighed against the risk of losing the mother during or after surgery due to inadequate resuscitation capacity in the face of sepsis or hypovolemic or hemorrhagic shock. In many cases, the mother dies from hypovolemic shock after a technically successful cesarean section with average blood loss simply because she cannot tolerate such loss. Such a situation may exist in women with severe chronic anemia due to malaria or other causes (e.g., malnutrition, hookworm, or other helminth infestation) where there has been time for the mother to compensate for a chronically low hemoglobin level (such as 4 or 5 mg/dl), but she is unable to sustain an average blood loss of 500 cc as the heart rate and output are already at the limits of their capacity. In these cases, blood pressure drops with slight changes in stroke volume, and there is no compensatory response. Performing spinal or general anesthesia on a woman in septic shock will often represent insurmountable stress. The clinician should understand that maternal outcome is primary and that some decisions that are absolutely not contemplated in high-resource settings must necessarily be implemented in such scenarios. The obstetric surgery algorithm includes acts that are different from those used in a well-resourced environment, such as assessing whether the mother can reasonably survive the anesthesia, stress, and blood loss of a normal C-section compared to her state of health. It may be reasonable to proceed with the surgery if the setting has all the characteristics to safely perform the surgery such as a skilled anesthetist and medical team and required equipment and blood products. If, on the other hand, she is in a facility without access to emergency resuscitation and blood transfusion, the wisest action could be to delay any surgery until the maternal condition improves or to transport the patient to a more equipped facility; such a decision could inevitably involve the loss of the fetus. In the case of fetal death and obstructed labor, performing a destructive fetal procedure to allow vaginal delivery and avoid major abdominal surgery may be an acceptable option in expert hands [37, 38]. Although the application of these procedures is a rare event and training in such practices is almost nonexistent in well-resourced environments, it would be advisable to carry out specific training considering multiple circumstances. Considering the low resources, abdominal surgery can be avoided in women with fetal death and placental abruption, and vaginal delivery can be performed safely without serious complications or loss of maternal life [39, 40]. In many resource-limited settings, the rate of uterine rupture is estimated to be much higher than in high-resource settings, possibly due to traditional practices that encourage the use of herbs and drugs to accelerate labor. Many of the decision-making problems mentioned above are not the ones that most physicians trained in high-resource settings usually face, so it would be necessary to be trained in high-level institutions before being employed in low-resource settings. This preparation may include participation in conferences, counseling by a mental health professional, simulated scenarios, and interviews with people with experience in this area. The staff should be closely monitored for signs of stress; demoralization; feelings of hopelessness, anger, and frustration with the local system; and PTSD (post-traumatic stress disorder), which can occur at any time during their stay.

3.1 C-section after obstructed labor

In some cases, a C-section after obstructed labor can cause high morbidity or mortality for the woman, so in case of fetal death and if a vaginal destructive procedure is possible, this may be the most advisable course of action. If the fetus is in a cephalic presentation, the skull can be shattered to remove the brain material, allowing the skull to collapse and stillbirth to happen. Although morally disturbing, in most cases, a vaginal delivery is preferable to a C-section. These women are particularly at risk of uterine atony and post-partum hemorrhage, so delivery should only be started in contexts where resuscitation is present; these women often have a history of recent or past infection and an increased risk of placental abruption: it is essential to start an antibiotic treatment and/or antithrombotic prophylaxis [41]. After childbirth and for several days of the puerperium, it is mandatory to perform a careful evaluation of the vagina and cervix to promptly diagnose vaginal, cervical, and bladder necrosis. All women who have had a long period of obstructed labor may need a bladder catheter for 5–7 days, and any fistula formation should be promptly diagnosed [41]. In those cases where there is a live fetus (or, in special circumstances, stillbirth) and an informed decision has been made to perform a C-section, there are some technical issues that deserve to be considered:

- Frequently, the baby will be deeply engaged in the pelvis due to prolonged labor;
- The lower uterine segment will be significantly thinned and can be retracted so that the bladder occupies its anatomical space;
- It is common for unsuspecting and inexperienced surgeons to perform an abdominal birth by dissecting the bladder during the creation of the uterine breach or the extraction of the baby.

The resulting damage can cause permanent damage to the urinary tract. The best way to avoid this situation is to initially disengage the fetal head vaginally, with a slight upward pressure, before starting the actual cesarean section. Disengagement may take a few minutes and is usually associated with a loud sucking sound and upward movement of the fetal head returning to the maternal pelvis. Overall, it is advisable to operate with the patient in a low lithotomy position to allow vaginal access during surgery; in addition, a midline incision should be made with extensive exposure of the lower uterine segment. The hysterotomy, after careful identification of the bladder, should be performed higher on the uterus than in an unobstructed labor; a narrow U-shaped incision, directed upward away from the uterine arteries, remains the preferable cutting mode. Before the extraction of the fetal head, an assistant can gently lift the head into the pelvis, to minimize trauma on the lower uterine segment and on the bladder. Uterine atony and postpartum hemorrhage may develop after the extraction, so it is necessary to administer oxytocin and start a uterine massage with manual compression of the myometrium. At the slightest sign of uterine atony and persistent hemorrhage, balloon tamponade (Bakri), compression sutures, and concomitant use of other uterotonic drugs should be resorted to immediately. In most low-resource settings, early recognition of bleeding and the aggressive use of methods to reduce blood loss are mandatory. In this setting, a fully dilated C-section can be performed even after a long labor, and such delays can cause further complications, including a longer hospital stay, increased risk of hemorrhage, the extension of the surgical incision with laceration of the vagina or uterine arteries, the development of lesions to the genitourinary and/or gastrointestinal tract, and the onset of postoperative fever [24]. In the case of extremely prolonged and hindered labor, necrosis of the cervix may develop with separation of the uterus and vagina, and it is almost always accompanied by the presence of a stillbirth, infection or sepsis, and extensive destruction of the bladder, usually at the level of the trine. At the same time, the risk of other complications, such as acute respiratory distress syndrome and pulmonary compromise, increases; it is advisable to transfer the patient to a reference center to avoid such occurrences. Hysterectomy may be the best option due to the likely presence of micro-abscesses in the damaged myometrial tissue, with such significant lesions and the high risk of uterine necrosis. Particular attention should be paid to the ureters to ensure their patency and integrity; in the event that the ureters were detached and no urological expertise is available, catheterization with ureteral stents and urine drainage in a sterile bag are used, while the patient is transported to a special department and undergoes definitive repair. It has recently been suggested that healthcare professionals should be trained to perform the symphysiotomy in all settings [42]. Symphysiotomy is an old operation in which the fibers of the pubic symphysis are partially divided to allow the separation of the symphysis and therefore the enlargement of the pelvic dimensions, in order to facilitate vaginal birth in the presence of cephalopelvic disproportion; this surgery can be performed under local anesthesia and does not require an operating room or advanced surgical skills [42, 43]. A recent review concluded that symphysiotomy can be a life-saving procedure in certain circumstances and that appropriate guidelines should be drawn up for the indications of this procedure [43].

3.2 C-section in obese women

Overweight and obesity (BMI 30–45) are more common than underweight in young women residing in both urban and rural areas of many countries with adequate economic resources. In the teaching hospital of the University of Nigeria, Enugu, from May 2008 to December 2010, there was an incidence of 12.4% of pathological maternal obesity [44]. Complication rates in obese women are similar in different parts of the world and include intra-partum and postoperative complications such as wound infection and endometritis, wound opening, hematoma, or seroma.

3.3 Myomectomy during C-section

Since access to blood products is insufficient in countries with limited resources and myomectomy is associated with an increase in blood loss, there is little experience in performing these two interventions in these settings. A study conducted in Accra, Ghana, comparing cesarean sections with and without myomectomy [45] enrolled 24 women, of whom 12 were with leiomyomas and 12 without. In women undergoing myomectomy within the cesarean section, the surgery duration was 11.25 minutes longer than that performed on women with a regular uterus; however, this difference was not statistically significant. There was comparable blood loss in the two groups, with an estimated mean of 392 mL in patients undergoing myomectomy versus 388 mL in patients in whom the procedure was not performed. In a systematic review of nine studies in women who underwent myomectomy during a cesarean section, there was a greater than 0.30 g/dL drop in hemoglobin in the myomectomy and cesarean group compared to the control group, but the difference was not found to be significant [46]. These data suggest that a cesarean section and myomectomy may be a reasonable option for those women (e.g., with anterior leiomyoma) who are potentially at risk for postoperative bleeding.

4. Conclusions

Even if a cesarean section is not always a complex surgical procedure, a complex set of elements and circumstances may compromise the outcome.

The surgical technique combined with the obstetric setting, clinical condition, and pregnancy pathology are factors to be taken into account before performing a cesarean section, to avoid major complications.

Medical formation and education on obstetric pathology are an important element that can change the clinical outcome.

Acronyms and abbreviations

C-section	cesarean section
CTG	cardiotocography
OR	odds ratio
TOLAC	trial of labor after a cesarean section
PROM	premature rupture of membranes
MAP	morbid attachment of the placenta
ICU	intensive care unit

Author details

Salvatore Felis[1*], Marta Fiamberti[2] and Chiara Peluffo[2]

1 Obstetric-Gynecology Department, IRCCS-San Martino Hospital, Genoa, Italy

2 Obstetric-Gynecology Department, IRCCS-San Martino Hospital, University of Genoa, Genoa, Italy

*Address all correspondence to: felissalvatore@libero.it

References

[1] Allen VM, O'Connell CM, Baskett TF. Maternal and perinatal morbidity of cesarean delivery at full cervical dilatation compared with cesarean delivery in the first stage of labour. BJOG. 2005;**112**(7):986-990

[2] Selo-Ojeme D, Sathiyathasan S, Fayyaz M. Cesarean delivery at full cervical dilatation versus cesarean delivery in the first stage of labour: Comparison of maternal and perinatal morbidity. Archives of Gynecology and Obstetrics. 2008;**278**(7):245-249

[3] Radha P, Tagore S, Rahman MF, Tee J. Maternal and perinatal morbidity after Cesarean delivery at full cervical dilatation. Singapore Medical Journal. 2012;**53**(10):655-658

[4] Ayres AW, Johnson TR, Hayashi R. Characteristics of fetal heart rate tracings prior to uterine rupture. International Journal of Gynaecology and Obstetrics. 2001;**74**(3):235-240

[5] Leung AS, Leung EK, Paul RH. Uterine rupture after previous cesarean delivery: Maternal and fetal consequences. American Journal of Obstetrics and Gynecology. 1993;**169**(4):945-950

[6] Landon MB, Hauth JC, Leveno KJ, Spong CY, Leindecker S, Varner MW, et al. Maternal and perinatal outcomes associated with a trial of labor after prior cesarean delivery. The New England Journal of Medicine. 2004;**351**(25):2581-2589

[7] Smith G, Pell J, Cameron A, Dobbie R. Risk of perinatal death associated with labor after previous cesarean delivery in uncomplicated term pregnancies. JAMA. 2002;**287**(20):2684-2690

[8] American College of Obstetricians and Gynecologists. ACOG practice Bulletin No. 115: vaginal birth after previous cesarean delivery. Obstetrics and Gynecology. 2010;**116**(2 Pt 1):450-463

[9] Akaba GO, Onafowokan O, Offiong RA, Omonua K, Ekele BA. Uterine rupture: Trends and feto-maternal outcome in a Nigerian teaching hospital. Nigerian Journal of Medicine. 2013;**22**(4):304-308

[10] World Health Organization. Estimated Obesity (BMI $\geq$ 30 kg/m^2) Prevalence, Females, Aged 15+. Available from: https://apps.who.int/infobase/Comparisons.aspx

[11] World Health Organization. BMI classification. 2016. Available from: http://apps.who.int/bmi/index.jsp?introPage= intro_3.html

[12] Weiss JL, Malone FD, Emig D, Ball RH, Nyberg DA, Comstock CH, et al. Obesity, obstetric complications and cesarean delivery rate: A population-based screening study. American Journal of Obstetrics and Gynecology. 2004;**190**(4):1091-1097

[13] Slavin VJ, Fenwick J, Gamble J. Pregnancy care and birth outcomes for women with moderate to super-extreme obesity. Women and Birth. 2013;**26**(3):179-184

[14] Chelmow D, Rodriguez EJ, Sabatini MM. Suture closure of subcutaneous fat and wound disruption after cesarean delivery: A meta-analysis. Obstetrics and Gynecology. 2004;**103**(5 Pt 1):974-980

[15] Coronado G, Marshall L, Schwartz S. Complications in pregnancy, labor, and

delivery with uterine leiomyomas: A population-based study. Obstetrics and Gynecology. 2000;**95**(5):764-769

[16] Klatsky PC, Tran ND, Caughey AB, Fujimoto VY. Fibroids and reproductive outcomes: A systematic literature review from conception to delivery. American Journal of Obstetrics and Gynecology. 2008;**198**(4):357-366

[17] Kaymak O, Ustunyurt E, Okyay R, Kalyoncu S, Mollamahmutoglu L. Myomectomy during cesarean section. International Journal of Gynaecology and Obstetrics. 2005;**89**(2):90-93

[18] Li H, Du J, Jin L, Shi Z, Liu M. Myomectomy during cesarean section. Acta Obstetricia et Gynecologica Scandinavica. 2009;**88**(2):183-186

[19] Morales KJ, Gordon MC, Bates GW. Postcesarean delivery adhesions associated with delayed delivery of infant. American Journal of Obstetrics and Gynecology. 2007;**196**(5):e461-e466

[20] Tulandi T, Al-Sannan B, Akbar G, Ziegler C, Miner L. Prospective study of intraabdominal adhesions among women of different races with or without keloids. American Journal of Obstetrics and Gynecology. 2011;**204**(2):e131-e134

[21] Malvasi A, Tinelli A, Guido M, Cavallotti C, Dell'Edera D, Zizza A, et al. Effect of avoiding bladder flap formation in cesarean section on repeat cesarean delivery. European Journal of Obstetrics, Gynecology, and Reproductive Biology. 2011;**159**(2):300-304

[22] Malvasi A, Tinelli A, Farine D, Rahimi S, Cavallotti C, Vergar D, et al. Effects of visceral peritoneal closure on scar formation at cesarean delivery. International Journal of Gynaecology and Obstetrics. 2009;**105**(2):131-135

[23] Lyell DJ, Caughey AB, Hu E, Blumenfeld Y, El-Sayed YY, Daniels K. Rectus muscle and visceral peritoneum closure at cesarean delivery and intraabdominal adhesions. American Journal of Obstetrics and Gynecology. 2012;**206**(6):e511-e515

[24] Cakir Gungor AN, Oguz S, Hacivelioglu S, Isik S, Uysal A, Gencer M, et al. Predictive value of striae gravidarum severity for intraperitoneal adhesions or uterine scar healing in patients with previous cesarean delivery. The Journal of Maternal-Fetal & Neonatal Medicine. 2013;**27**(13):1312-1315

[25] Pandit SN, Khan RJ. Surgical techniques for performing cesarean section including CS at full dilatation. Best Practice & Research. Clinical Obstetrics & Gynaecology. 2013;**27**(2):179-195

[26] Mhyre JM, Tsen LC, Einav S, Kuklina EV, Leffert LR, Bateman BT. Cardiac arrest during hospitalization for delivery in the United States, 1998-2011. Anesthesiology. 2014;**120**(4):810-818

[27] Jeejeebhoy FM, Zelop CM, Windrim R, Carvalho JC, Dorian P, Morrison LJ. Management of cardiac arrest in pregnancy: A systematic review. Resuscitation. 2011;**82**(7):801-809

[28] Morrison LJ, Deakin CD, Morley PT, Callaway CW, Kerber RE, Kronick SL, et al. Part 8: Advanced life support: 2010 International consensus on cardiopulmonary resuscitation and emergency cardiovascular care science with treatment recommendations. Circulation. 2010;**122**(16 Suppl. 2):S345-S421

[29] Katz VL. Perimortem cesarean delivery: Its role in maternal mortality. Seminars in Perinatology. 2012;**36**(1):68-72

[30] O'Leary JL, O'Leary JA. Uterine artery ligation in the control of

intractable postpartum hemorrhage. American Journal of Obstetrics and Gynecology. 1966;**94**(7):920-924

[31] AbdRabbo SA. Stepwise uterine devascularization: A novel technique for management of uncontrolled postpartum hemorrhage with preservation of the uterus. American Journal of Obstetrics and Gynecology. 1994;**171**(3):694-700

[32] Belfort MA, Zimmerman J, Schemmer G, Oldroyd R, Smilanich R, Pearce M. Aortic compression and cross clamping in a case of placenta percreta and amniotic fluid embolism: A case report. AJP Reports. 2011;**1**(1):33-36

[33] Sovik E, Stokkeland P, Storm BS, Asheim P, Bolas O. The use of aortic occlusion balloon catheter without fluoroscopy for life-threatening post-partum haemorrhage. Acta Anaesthesiologica Scandinavica. 2012;**56**(3):388-393

[34] Chandraharan E, Rao S, Belli AM, Arulkumaran S. The Triple-P procedure as a conservative surgical alternative to peripartum hysterectomy for placenta percreta. International Journal of Gynaecology and Obstetrics. 2012;**117**(2):191-194

[35] Dildy GA, Scott JR, Saffer CS, Belfort MA. An effective pressure pack for severe pelvic hemorrhage. Obstetrics and Gynecology. 2006;**108**(5):1222-1226

[36] Charoenkwan K. Effective use of the Bakri postpartum balloon for posthysterectomy pelvic floor hemorrhage. American Journal of Obstetrics and Gynecology. 2014;**210**(6):e581-e583

[37] Lawson J. Embryotomy for obstructed labour. Tropical Doctor. 1974;**4**(4):188-191

[38] Smale LE. Destructive operations on the fetus: Review of literature and application in 10 cases of neglected dystocia. American Journal of Obstetrics and Gynecology. 1974;**119**(3):369-374

[39] Belfort M. A new instrument for the delivery of the impacted dead fetus. Tropical Doctor. 1988;**18**(4):180-182

[40] Belfort M, Moore P. The use of a cephalic perforator for delivery of the dead fetus in cases of severe abruptio placentae. South African Medical Journal. 1990;**77**:80-82

[41] Creanga AA, Genadry RR. Obstetric fistulas: A clinical review. International Journal of Gynaecology and Obstetrics. 2007;**99**(Suppl. 1):S40-S46

[42] Monjok E, Okokon IB, Opiah MM, Ingwu JA, Ekabua JE, Essien EJ. Obstructed labour in resource-poor settings: The need for revival of symphysiotomy in Nigeria. African Journal of Reproductive Health. 2012;**16**(3):94-101

[43] Hofmeyr GJ, Shweni PM. Symphysiotomy for feto-pelvic disproportion. Cochrane Database of Systematic Reviews. 2012;**10**: CD005299

[44] Okafor UV, Efetie ER, Nwoke O, Okezie O, Umeh U. Anaesthetic and obstetric challenges of morbid obesity in cesarean deliveries: A study in South-eastern Nigeria. African Health Sciences. 2012;**12**(1):54-57

[45] Kwawukume E. Myomectomy during cesarean section. International Journal of Gynaecology and Obstetrics. 2002;**76**(2):183-184

[46] Song D, Zhang W, Chames MC, Guo J. Myomectomy during cesarean delivery. International Journal of Gynaecology and Obstetrics. 2013;**121**(3):208-213

Section 5

Pregnancy Assesment, Cardiotocografy, Doppler Ultrasound and Fetal Ultrasound

Chapter 7

Patient Blood Management in Cesarean Section

Pablo Santillán Roldan, Andrés Cepeda Mora, Pablo Armas Cruz, Andres Sarmiento Benavides, María Victoria Iturralde Arcos, Juan Carlos Jacome Sayay, Elisa Aucapiña Chocho and María Isabel Jara Jimbo

Abstract

Worldwide, every minute a woman dies due to complications during pregnancy, obstetric hemorrhage being the leading cause. However, most of these deaths are preventable with prompt recognition and management. The main objective of its management in the initial phase of resuscitation is to aggressively optimize macro and microhemodynamic parameters by ensuring effective resuscitation. Patient blood management (PBM) consists in the timely application of evidence-based medical and surgical procedures aimed at maintaining hemoglobin concentration, optimizing hemostasis and minimizing blood loss to improve patient outcome, all of these based in three pillars: endogenous erythropoiesis, platelet and coagulation factors function and physiological reserve of anemia. PBM consider various strategies to reach the main goal, including transfusional, non-transfusional and surgical measures. At preoperative period the prevention and treatment of anemia is the corner stone of the PBM guideline. Once at the operating room the fluid management, uterotonic and pro-coagulant drugs, fibrinogen and blood products transfusion play a key role and surgical techniques have to be done if the patient life is threatened. Manage postpartum anemia by appropriate iron administration. Optimize the patient's physiological response to anemia, treat infections and maximize oxygen delivery to minimize transfusions if they are not strictly necessary.

Keywords: obstetric hemorrhages, massive transfusion, pregnancy Anemia, fibrinogen, blood management

1. Introduction

Worldwide, every minute, a woman dies due to complications during pregnancy, obstetric hemorrhage being the leading cause; however, most of these deaths are preventable. Hypovolemic shock is the main consequence of obstetric hemorrhage. Obstetric hemorrhage is one of the five leading causes of maternal mortality in both high-resource countries and resource-limited countries, although the absolute risk of death from obstetric hemorrhage is much lower in the former [1–3].

Prompt recognition, availability of appropriate resources, and adequate responses are critical to preventing mortality and severe maternal morbidity [1–3].

Normally, hemostasis occurs with the separation of the placenta, and control of uterine bleeding is done through a combination of two mechanisms: [4].

- Mechanical hemostasis, whereby contraction of the myometrium compresses the blood vessels supplying the placental bed, resulting in a severe reduction in blood flow [4].

- Local thrombosis, by the presence or release of local decidual hemostatic factors (tissue factor and plasminogen activator inhibitor type 1) and systemic coagulation factors (platelets, circulating coagulation factors), leading to thrombosis of damaged blood vessels supplying the placental bed, resulting in severe reduction of blood flow [4].

Once obstetric bleeding occurs, the goals of treatment are to aggressively optimize macro and microhemodynamic parameters by ensuring effective resuscitation and timely replacement of blood products in addition to subsequent surgical management.

Patient blood management (PBM) consists of the timely application of evidence-based medical and surgical procedures aimed at maintaining hemoglobin concentration, optimizing hemostasis, and minimizing blood loss to improve patient outcome, all of these based on three pillars: endogenous erythropoiesis, platelet & coagulation factor functions, and physiological reserve of anemia, guided by the obstetric hemorrhage scenario. The multidisciplinary approach plays a key role even from preoperative to postoperative period, improving outcomes and reducing morbi-mortality in this population and hospitalization length and costs.

PBM considers various strategies to reach the main goal, including transfusional, non-transfusional, and surgical measures. In the preoperative period, the prevention and prompt treatment of anemia is one of the cornerstones of the PBM guideline; despite all the physiological changes during pregnancy, every single pregnant woman has an increased risk for a major bleeding due to several risk factors specific to pregnancy and each patient. Once at the operating room, leading causes for postpartum hemorrhage are widely described, so it is important that both the gynecologist and the anesthesiologist be prepared to solve the emergency, the fluid management, uterotonic and pro-coagulant drugs, fibrinogen, and, finally, blood product transfusion with all the concerns about it. Surgical techniques like B-lynch, Hayman technique, or others more advance like postpartum hysterectomy have to be used if the patient's life is threatened [5].

Manage postpartum anemia by appropriate iron administration. Optimize the patient's physiological response to anemia, treat infections, and maximize oxygen delivery to minimize transfusions if they are not strictly necessary.

2. First Pilar: enlargement of red blood cell mass

During pregnancy, physiological changes take place and prepare the woman in several ways, especially for the delivery moment and prevention of blood loss at this time. One of them is the hematological system, where maternal plasma volume expansion reaches a net increase of approximately 50% by 34 weeks' gestation. Red blood cells rise to 30% above the pre-pregnancy level at term due to an increased concentration of erythropoietin and the erythropoietic effect of progesterone, prolactin, and placental lactoge [5, 6].

The difference in the increase in blood elements results in hemodilution, which is known as physiologic anemia of pregnancy. Despite the hemodilution, the rheological changes ensure enough oxygen delivery, better placental perfusion, less risk for thrombosis, despite the bleeding that occurs with childbirth, the objectives being to improve the main outcome of the first pillar [5, 6].

At the same time, there is a substantial increase of the coagulation factors I, VII, VIII, IX, X, and XII and von Willebrand factor. Furthermore, there is a decrease of Factor XI and XIII and a physiologic decrease of protein S, while F II and V do not change, resulting in an accelerated but compensated intravascular coagulation state [6].

The main objective of patient blood management strategies in pregnancy is to prevent postpartum hemorrhage (PPH) and decrease morbi-mortality associated with blood products transfusion. Thus, the first step is to recognize risk factors, so women with previous PPH in the last pregnancy, pre-existing anemia, prior cesarean section, multiple gestations, uterine fibroma, preeclampsia, obesity, chorioamnionitis, and fetal macrosomia are at increased risk for PPH [7, 8].

However, almost 61% of women with PPH do not have a risk factor, excluding maternal age and cesarean section. Therefore, we have to consider that all pregnant women have a considerable risk for PPH [7, 8].

From all of the possible risk factors, anemia and iron deficiency are susceptible to modification, and this is where the first pillar of the PBM could be specifically implemented. Pregnant women are the only patients in whom we can detect iron deficiency and anemia long before a potential blood loss at delivery [5].

Anemia affects approximately 40% of pregnant women worldwide with iron deficiency as main cause. Anemia has been associated with several complications like the need for increased health care requirements, intensive care for both the mother and neonate, higher rates of preeclampsia, higher rates of induction of labor, cesarean delivery, blood transfusion and higher rates of infectious disease for both mother and newborn, all of these anemia severity – dependent, increasing maternal y perinatal morbidity and mortality [7, 9, 10].

Anemia treatment has the potential to improve outcomes for affected women and their fetuses and neonates and minimize the illness burden and cost due to this common disease [9].

Once the diagnosis of anemia is done, we have to evaluate the cause of the disease, starting with iron metabolism analysis because it is responsible for 60% of anemia cases. In pregnancy, iron requirement increases considerably, and mother's stores cannot fulfill this need most of the time. Therefore, all guidelines of obstetric care recommend a complete hematological investigation when a low hemoglobin value is detected including transferrin level, iron saturation and supplementation with iron o B12 if needed [5, 10].

Iron metabolism evaluation must be done with ferritin screening (30 – 100 ng/ml as normal cutoff) where values below 30 ng/ml mean clear iron deficiency, even with normal hemoglobin, as it is the best and most practical marker for iron store evaluation. Nevertheless, serum ferritin is also an acute-phase protein, so this value increases during infectious or inflammatory episodes. It is recommended to measure the C – reactive Protein (CRP) levels with normal ferritin in case of low Hb in inflammatory situations [5, 10, 11].

Other markers we can evaluate for iron deficiency are red cell distribution width (RDW) and mean corpuscular hemoglobin (MHC). Transferrin saturation rate is a marker that shows us the percentage of iron binding sites that are occupied. The normal values are between 20 and 50%, where levels below 20% mean iron deficiency [5, 10].

WHO recommends routine iron supplementation for every pregnant woman, especially in low-income countries, to prevent iron deficiency without anemia and iron deficiency with anemia with 30 – 60 mg/day of oral iron. In cases of mild or moderate anemia, it is advised to have an iron substitution of 160 – 200 mg/day. Iron supplementation usually has gastrointestinal side effects; when it is administrated during the first trimester, it can worsen nausea or gestational emesis, gastric pain, or constipation. Intravenous iron is indicated when there is intolerance to oral iron preparations or when Hb does not increase appropriately (less than 1 g/dl within 14 days) or when there is severe anemia during the third trimester or progressive anemia or if a rapid treatment is needed [5, 10, 11].

The optimal duration of iron deficiency treatment is 6–8 weeks with periodical Hb and serum ferritin screening every 4 weeks [10, 11].

3. Second Pillar: Minimization of bleeding and targeted transfusion therapy

After optimizing the volume of bleeding, the second pillar of management consists of minimizing blood loss, for which it is necessary to identify the forecast of surgical bleeding; adequate management of antiplatelet agents and anticoagulants; optimal anesthetic techniques to minimize bleeding; monitoring of the bleeding and coagulopathy; and devising an anesthetic plan.

According to the Spanish Scientific Society of Anesthesiology, Resuscitation and Pain Treatment, in order to achieve an efficient anesthetic plan, the anesthesiologist is required to use a multimodal approach within their perioperative management, including the following:

- Hypotensive resuscitation
- Use of antifibrinolytics
- Proper use of hemostatic agents

Hemostatic management of intraoperative bleeding requires careful control of coagulation.

4. Hypotensive resuscitation

Its fundamental objective is based on lowering blood pressure until definitive hemostasis and adequate tissue perfusion are achieved [12].

Their approach narrows to using small volumes of crystalloids as they are less likely to create dilutional coagulopathy, and lower blood pressure is less likely to break up or fragment the already formed clot; however, when large volumes of fluid are administered, this can initiate dilution of coagulation factors, resulting in impaired coagulation and coagulopathy [12].

A cohort study showed that lower fluid administration showed fewer signs of shock and less blood product administration, as fibrinogen, hemoglobin, hematocrit, and platelet concentrations decreased during increased fluid administration, whereas PT and aPTT were more prolonged [13].

Therefore, the most recent studies have reported that resuscitation with >4 L of fluids is associated with subsequent bleeding and more adverse maternal outcomes [14]. Hypoperfusion can be tolerated for short periods of time and may decrease the volume of overall hemorrhage [12].

During hemorrhagic shock, the endothelial glycocalyx is thinned, and administration of crystalloids exacerbates this state, leading to more fluid extravasation and general volume depletion, leading to worsening bleeding [12].

5. Drugs used for intraoperative bleeding administration

Use of synthetic antifibrinolytic agents, such as epsilon-aminocaproic acid (EACA) or tranexamic acid, reduces blood loss and blood transfusion during cardiac procedures and is indicated for blood conservation (Class I, Level A) [15]. The main function of these components is to limit clot formation and ensure adequate blood flow, establishing a dynamic balance with the coagulation system [16].

6. Tranexamic acid

Initially, its use was limited to the treatment of obstetric hemorrhages and hemophiliac patients. Subsequently, it was progressively extended to cardiac surgery and the rest of its current indications [16].

Aminocaproic acid are lysine analogs that reversibly inhibit fibrinolysis by binding to lysine binding sites on plasminogen, limiting plasmin activation, which cleaves fibrin strands [17].

A Cochrane review of the effectiveness and safety of tranexamic acid (TXA), which identified 51 studies of antifibrinolytics, found that TXA produced an RR of RBC transfusion of 0·61 (95 percent ci 0·53 to 0·70) and concluded that "lysine analogues are effective in reducing blood loss during and after surgery, and appear to be free of serious adverse effects" [17].

Dosage and dosing schedules vary depending on the clinical setting, but a 1 g dose is sufficient for most adults, with no evidence to support the use of high doses [16]. CRASH-2 (Clinical Randomization Trial of an Antifibrinolytic in significant bleeding) showed that early administration of 1 g of tranexamic acid (within 3 hours of traumatic injury) followed by a 1 g infusion over 8 hours significantly reduced the risk of death from bleeding and all-cause mortality in traumatic bleeding [17].

In cardiac interventions, the dose range was 2.5 mg/kg to 100 mg/kg, and for the maintenance dose, it was 0.25 mg/kg/h to 4.0 mg/kg/h, over 1 to 12 hours. These variations were also observed in non-cardiac surgery [18].

A meta-analysis showed that TXA significantly reduced blood loss compared with placebo; of the studies that reported the number of transfusions, administration of tranexamic acid was reported to reduce an average of 1.12 units compared with placebo and was not associated with an increase in morbidity or mortality [18].

Based on the CRASH 2 trial, CRASH 3 trial and WOMAN trial results TXA is the first choice for antifibrinolytic therapy in any hemorrhagic scenario due it effectiveness and cost/benefits evaluation [18].

The 2017 WHO recommendation on tranexamic acid for the treatment of obstetric hemorrhage states that tranexamic acid should be recognized as a life-saving intervention and readily available for the management of PPH in settings where emergency obstetric care is provided, regardless of the level of medical care system resources [19].

A meta-analysis of two trials showed that immediate treatment improved survival by >70%, and thereafter, the survival benefit decreased by 10% for each 15 min delay in treatment until 3 h, after which there was no benefit [20].

In an effort to administer TXA as early as possible, in a pre-hospital setting, its use is now supported by UK ambulance services, current research is evaluating alternative dosages and formulations, including intramuscular TXA, which appears more feasible for timely administration in emergencies [20].

7. Other hemostatic agents

7.1 Prothrombin complex concentrate

PCCs or prothrombin complex concentrates are plasma-derived compounds containing highly purified vitamin K-dependent coagulation factors (II, VII, IX, and X) with hemostatic activity [21].

Originally, the main indication for PCC was the reversal of the effect of vitamin K antagonists; however, they are now also used to treat congenital or acquired conditions such as factor II or factor X deficiencies and are useful in the treatment of massive traumatic bleeding [22].

Systematic reviews have identified little scientific evidence on the use of PCC in adult patients with major bleeding; although the use of PCC is safe and recommended for urgent cases of reversal of the effect of vitamin K antagonists, there is currently limited evidence to support its use in the management of major bleeding unrelated to vitamin K antagonists [20].

In addition to a Cochrane review published on PCC for patients with vitamin K antagonists undergoing emergency surgery, PCCs appear to have a very safe profil with a minimal thromboembolic risk in these cases. One report has described the beneficial use of PCC in PPH in one patient with a non-hereditary coagulation deficiency [19].

In a retrospective study of 14 obstetric cases with disseminated intravascular coagulation (DIC), the use of PCCs failed to alter the outcome, which is why the use of PCCs cannot be considered a part of standard clinical practice for obstetric hemorrhage [20].

Efficacy in INR correction is also an advantage of prothrombin complex concentrates over fresh frozen plasma [21]. A retrospective study compared both treatments in patients with intracranial hemorrhage associated with anticoagulation and demonstrated that subjects treated with prothrombin complex concentrates had an average decrease in INR from 2.83 to 1.22 in 4.8 hours vs. a decrease from 2.97 to 1.74 in 7.3 hours in those who received fresh frozen plasma, that is, 4 to 5 times longer and less effective, with a statistically significant difference ($p \leq 0.001$) [21].

A single 40 mL (1000 IU) dose of PCC is functionally equivalent to the adult FFP dose of 10 to 15 mL/kg, or four to five plasma quantity units or 1000 mL volume, all classes of PCC include factors II, IX, and X, whereas the four-factor PCC also contains clinically relevant factor VII.

Some authors suggest a dose of 25–30 IU/kg, supported by the results of an open clinical study, without random distribution, carried out in patients with high INR (between 8.9 and 18 and greater than 20) [21].

In Canada, the approved PCC indications include rapid reversal of vitamin K deficiency in patients with severe bleeding or need for emergency surgery within 6 hours, but it is not recommended for surgery that may get delayed 6 to 12 hours, since in PCC anticoagulant reversal, its effect is temporary due to the short half - life of factor VII factor, which falls after 6 hours [23].

Consequently, intravenous administration with 10 mg of vitamin K with PCC is recommended to activate existing coagulation factors and maintain the reversal effect, as vitamin K1 reaches clinical effect within 6 hours by which PCC effects begin to weaken [23].

The administration of higher doses of prothrombin complex concentrates has been described in relation to the degree of INR prolongation.

It is not recommended to pass a maximum dose of PCC of 3000 IU (120 mL).

7.2 Fibrinogen concentrate

Fibrinogen, also called Factor I, is a blood plasma protein produced by the liver that plays a key role in hemostasis. It is the coagulation factor with the highest plasma concentration, between 150 and 400 mg/dl [24].

In its mechanism of action we have, it acts in both primary and secondary hemostasis; its soluble form serves to bind to activated platelets, forming bridges between them after binding to the glycoprotein IIb -IIIa receptor on its surface, contributing to the platelet aggregation and platelet plug formation during primary hemostasis; subsequently, fibrinogen is converted to fibrin monomers, which are polymerized, with the help of factor XIIIa, to an insoluble form (fibrin) that stabilizes the platelet plug and provides a firm mesh for clot propagation during secondary hemostasis [24].

Hypofibrinogenemia as a result of blood loss, factor consumption, or hemodilution is associated with poor patient outcomes and increased mortality in trauma patients [25]. The fibrinogen concentration upon arrival at the hospital may vary depending on the individual, patient factors; for example, low fibrinogen levels have been associated with young age, male gender, long time since injury, low base excess, and high injury severity score [25].

Starting INR	Minimum dose (IU/kg)	Maximum dose (IU/kg)
2.0–2.5	22.5	32.5
2.5–3.0	32.5	40
3.0–3.5	40	47.5
> 3.5		47.5

There are several techniques available to determine the fibrinogen concentration; the Clauss technique is recommended for diagnostic purposes or when decisions regarding the clinical management of patients with hemorrhage must be made [18]. The determination of FIBTEM with ROTEM or Functional Fibrinogen in TEG allows rapid detection of changes in fibrinogen levels in trauma patients. In this regard, it has been confirmed that the determination of fibrinogen using the FIBTEM test in ROTEM® is closely related to the values obtained with the Clauss method [18].

Fresh frozen plasma or FFP, cryoprecipitate, and human fibrinogen concentrate are available options for fibrinogen replacement. They contain approximately 2.5, 15, and 20 g/L of fibrinogen, respectively. Both FFP and cryoprecipitate require thawing and crossmatching prior to infusion, with known potential transfusion-related complications and risks. Cryoprecipitate is still not available in many European countries [22].

FIBTEM amplitude at 10 min from onset of clot formation (FIBTEMA10) correlates with fibrinogen concentration and thus allows early identification of fibrinogen deficiency. FIBTEMA10 < 7 mm has been suggested as a trigger for fibrinogen replacement with the aim of raising FIBTEMA10 to at least 10 mm during ongoing bleeding [18].

In maternity patients, fibrinogen levels rise to an average of 5–6 g/L at term (compared to nonpregnant levels of 2.0–4.5 g/L). Low fibrinogen levels are an independent risk factor for the development of severe PPH, with a study that showed levels below 2 g/L with a 100% positive predictive value for the development of severe PPH [14].

In Australia, the most common way to increase plasma fibrinogen levels is to transfuse cryoprecipitate. This plasma-derived blood product contains high levels of fibrinogen, factor VIII, von Willebrand factor, factor XIII, and fibronectin. To provide a 3 to 4 g dose of fibrinogen, about 8 to 10 bags (typically 30 to 40 mL), which require thawing [14].

Fibrinogen concentrate is available as a lyophilized powder in 1- or 2-gram vials, and the protein is reconstituted with 50 or 100 mL, respectively, of sterile water. The final concentration, therefore, is 2 g/100 ml. It can be kept at room temperature, with a durability of 5 years [24].

Pharmacokinetic studies in patients with congenital afibrinogenemia show that substitution of 1 mg/kg of fibrinogen increases the plasma concentration by around 1.38–1.5 mg/dl, with a volume of distribution of 90–100 ml/kg [24]. The infusion rate should not exceed 5 ml/min (1 g/10 min), although cases have been described with a much higher transfusion rate without thrombus formation being observed in the vessel [24].

Fibrinogen concentrate prevents adverse effects associated with allogeneic blood products, including transfusion-related acute lung injury and incompatibility [20].

The administration of CCP together with factor XIII and fibrinogen (guided by the results of TEM) more effectively reversed the associated coagulopathy and the need for massive transfusion than conventional plasma therapy, without observable differences in the development of multi-organ failure, in hospital stay or mortality [14].

7.3 Clot stability and FXIII (Fibrin Stabilizer)

FXIII is known to be an essential contributor to clot strength through its ability to cross-link and stabilize fibrin; however, most bleeding management guidelines currently do not include measurement and subsequent supplementation of FXIII [25].

Clot instability due to FXIII deficiency has been identified in some cases by ROTEM; in the neurosurgical setting, a postoperative FXIII level < 60% was found to be an independent risk factor for postoperative ICH [14].

In cases of bleeding and low FXIII activity (e.g., <30%), the administration of FXIII concentrate (30 IU/kg) is suggested, [25] although other studies recommend its use at a dose of 20 IU/kg of ideal weight, either by cryoprecipitates or plasma [26].

7.4 Activated recombinant human factor VII (rhFVIIa)

Recombinant human factor VIIa (rhFVIIa) is a tissue factor, activated prohemostatic agent, the efficacy of rhVIIa has been demonstrated in nonrandomized studies in severe postpartum hemorrhage. The risk of thromboembolic complications has not been systematically investigated; it requires correction of hypothermia, acidosis, fibrinogen levels, and anemia; therefore, if bleeding could not be controlled by other measures, rhFVIIa could reduce the need for second-line therapies [13].

In a prospective cohort study with 22 patients with severe PPH, rhVIIa contributed to PPH control, and hysterectomy was avoided, and in life-threatening PPH, rFVIIa administration could be used; however, this should not replace or postpone vital interventions, but it should be noted that patients should be monitored for thromboembolism, especially if rhVIIa is administered in combination with tranexamic acid [13].

8. Administration of blood products

8.1 Packed red blood cells

There is a lack of evidence to support the benefit of blood transfusions, specifically in the case of hemodynamically stable patients undergoing elective surgery. Furthermore, it is an independent risk factor for adverse effects [18].

It is recommended to base its administration on clinical (blood pressure, heart rate) and biological (lactate, base excess) parameters, with a hemoglobin target of 8 g/dl, considering figures >9 g/dl for risk patients (heart disease). ischemic, cardiac surgery, etc.) considering the transfusion of red blood cells in most patients only when the Hb concentration is less than 7 g/ dL [26].

The Transfusion Requirements in Septic Shock (TRISS) trial showed that severely ill patients with septic shock could safely benefit from an Hb threshold of 7 g/dL132. Furthermore, an RCT of upper gastrointestinal bleeding in 921 patients, of whom a third were admitted with signs of hypovolemic shock (systolic BP <100 mmHg), demonstrated that an Hb threshold of 7 g/dl was safe and increased survival at 45 days when applied from the earliest phase [19].

The indication for blood transfusion should be more restrictive without fixed criteria for red blood cell transfusions; Hb below 6 g/dl generally requires a transfusion of 1 RGC, while this is rarely the case in a hemodynamically stable situation with an Hb of 8 g/dL or higher. Between 6 and 8 g/ dL, the indication for transfusion should be more restrictive, depending on the clinical situation and the patient's symptoms, since the best recommendation is to avoid the transfusion of packed red blood cells [13].

8.2 Fresh frozen plasma

Fresh frozen plasma (FFP) has limited clotting capacity and is inferior to fibrinogen concentrate for the treatment of hypofibrinogenemia. As a colloidal infusion, FFP is given for volume resuscitation in situations with severe hypovolemia and concomitant coagulopathy [13].

We suggest transfusing a standard dose of plasma (15–20 mL/kg) in ongoing severe PPH guided by abnormal coagulation tests (e.g., prolonged TEG time) [19].

From an empirical point of view, the administration of fresh plasma should be started after the loss of 1–1.5 blood volumes. During massive hemorrhage, early administration of fresh plasma is recommended to prevent or treat coagulopathy, taking into account that thawing of FFP requires a long time, and therefore, timely organization of FFP is recommended [26].

The use of large volumes of fresh plasma can lead to transfusion-associated circulatory overload (TACO), probably the most common complication today, while others, such as acute respiratory distress syndrome (ARDS), lung injury related to transfusion (TRALI), and hemolytic reactions, are exceptional. PFC should not be used prior to a procedure to correct mild to moderate elevated INR (less than 2.0) [26].

8.3 Platelet concentrate

Platelets play a key role in hemostasis and clot formation. Although very few trauma patients have low platelet counts on admission, it is very likely that platelet deficiency will develop over time depending on treatment [13]. The insufficient number of platelets is characterized by EXTEMCA10 < 40 mm (but normal FIBTEM amplitude) and low platelets (<50,000/L), which will indicate the need for administration of platelet concentrate [25].

Platelet transfusions have been considered a safe and potentially effective intervention in major bleeding; the results of the PATCH trial demonstrated that platelet transfusion increased the risk of death in patients receiving antiplatelet therapy (mainly aspirin) and presenting with acute spontaneous intracerebral hemorrhage (stroke), although methodological limitations have been described [20].

There are no solid data on the number of platelets necessary to guarantee primary hemostasis in different clinical situations, so its administration is also based on the severity of the bleeding and the particular circumstances that caused the massive bleeding. It is recommended to maintain a platelet count >50 × 109/l in patients with active bleeding, and it is suggested to increase it to 75–100 × 109/l in situations of uncontrolled massive bleeding or head trauma [26].

Long-term prophylactic platelet transfusions should be avoided due to the risk of complications (including alloimmunization and platelet refractoriness) [18].

8.4 Improvement of platelet function: desmopressin

Desmopressin, 1-desamino-8-D-arginine vasopressin (DDAVP) is a synthetic analog of the antidiuretic pituitary hormone arginine vasopressin. In vivo, it causes an increase in factor VIII levels and stimulates the release of von Willebrand factor from endothelial cells, which promotes platelet adhesion to wound sites. DDAVP can be used to correct the anti-hemostatic effect of aspirin and clopidogrel and can also be applied as part of the treatment for platelet dysfunction or von Willebrand's disease and also as an alternative use for enhancement of platelet increase [22].

8.5 Cryoprecipitates

Cryoprecipitate is a high molecular weight protein concentrate containing coagulation factors VIII and XIII and von Willebrand, together with fibronectin and platelet microparticles. It is obtained in blood banks from a PFC unit by thawing it at low temperature (1–6°C). The precipitated proteins are separated by centrifugation, and the supernatant is removed, leaving the insoluble precipitate, which is later resuspended in 5–20 ml of plasma that is then frozen again and stored at −18°C. Each unit of cryoprecipitate is generally collected in bags *(pool)* of five units [24].

Mortality and the number of RGC units transfused in 24 h are higher in patients who receive cryoprecipitate transfusions compared to those who do not. Mortality at

30 days was higher in patients who received cryoprecipitate transfusions compared with those who did not [12].

The number of cryoprecipitates transfused was higher in those who received cryoprecipitate transfusions compared to those who did not receive cryoprecipitate. No evidence was found for the critical impact parameters [18].

Consider transfusing cryoprecipitates in patients without major bleeding who have the following:

clinically significant bleeding

Fibrinogen levels below 2 g/l

9. Third Pillar:optimizing postoperative/postpartum treatment of anemia

Apart from the identification and appropriate action in each phase of obstetric hemorrhage, another fundamental pillar in the management of severe primary obstetric hemorrhage is the assessment with laboratory tests that include: blood biometrics, fibrinogen, coagulation studies, and lactate and base deficit (arterial blood gases) as they are tools to evaluate systemic tissue perfusion and are called **"optimal laboratory,"** since hemoglobin and hematocrit do not accurately reflect the amount of blood lost acutely [27].

Within coagulation studies should be requested fibrinogen concentration, prothrombin time, and activated partial thromboplastin time; this coagulation panel should be repeated every 30 to 60 minutes to observe trends until bleeding is controlled; coagulation studies are usually normal in the early stages of bleeding, but they can be abnormal when comorbidities exist, such as placental abruption, liver disease, stillbirth, sepsis, or amniotic fluid embolism. Eventually, significant bleeding without replacement of clotting factors will result in clotting abnormalities [27].

Fibrinogen is a cable point in the assessment of hemostasis since it falls to critically low levels before other clotting factors during a hemorrhage, so the level of fibrinogen is the most sensitive indicator of a significant loss of blood in progress, since its fall is related to the loss of fibrinogen through bleeding, increased fibrinolytic activity, and hemodilution secondary to fluids administered to maintain blood pressure during initial resuscitation, so it can be used to guide the aggressiveness of treatment [28, 29]. The normal level of fibrinogen in a full-term pregnancy is 350 to 650 mg/dl, which is almost twice that of a non-pregnant woman (200 to 400 mg/dl); a low level of fibrinogen (less than 200 mg/dL) is a predictor of major bleeding that is associated with the need for transfusion of multiple units of blood and blood products, the need for surgical treatment of bleeding, and increased maternal morbidity and mortality [30, 31].

Another pillar of the assessment is viscoelastic tests such as thromboelastography (TEG) and rotational thromboelastometry (ROTEM), which are very useful when available, as they are useful to guide the administration therapy of plasma and other coagulation products. These tests provide a global assessment of complete hemostasis (time to clot development, clot stabilization/resistance, and clot dissolution) and can be performed at the bedside, so results are available within minutes. The results are useful for choosing only the transfusion-specific blood components that a patient requires and evaluating the efficacy of the interventions performed [32, 33]. The use of viscoelastic testing has led to fibrinogen replacement much earlier than with standard coagulation tests, and this early and aggressive fibrinogen replacement is thought to prevent severe coagulopathy and reduce maternal morbidity and mortality [33].

Once the initial treatment was established, bleeding control was achieved, and optimal laboratory tests were run; the objectives in the patient after obstetric hemorrhage are: [26].

- Hemoglobin>7.5 g/dL
- Platelets >50,000/mm^3
- Fibrinogen >200 mg/dL
- Prothrombin time less than 1.5 times the control value
- Activated partial thromboplastin time less than 1.5 times the control value

The first objective is to obtain a hemoglobin of 7.5 g/dl; to make the corrections, we must remember that most guides recommend continuing to transfuse patients with hemoglobin values lower than 7.5 to 8 g/dl; however, our recommendation is to maintain a hemoglobin level of at least 8 g/dl after transfusion, since values below this level may be associated with hemostasis altered by lower platelet adhesion and high blood velocity, as well as an increased likelihood of myocardial ischemia; however, a common practice is to maintain blood transfusion in any patient with hemoglobin less than 7 g/dl, regardless of whether it is symptomatic or not, and to transfuse symptomatic patients with a hemoglobin value <8 g/dL [33].

Iron supplements are also recommended because the amount of iron lost is not completely replaced with transfused blood. Oral supplements are an option, and single-dose parenteral iron therapy is another option. The advantages of parenteral iron are that hemoglobin levels increase faster, anemia symptoms improve earlier, and less gastric discomfort occurs compared to oral therapy. However, most women with mild to moderate anemia resolve anemia quickly enough with oral iron, and this measure is inexpensive and convenient [33].

Erythropoietin may increase the rate of recovery to normal hemoglobin levels; however, it does not have an immediate effect and has not been shown to reduce transfusion requirements after bleeding, is also no more effective than iron therapy in this setting, and is expensive, so its use is not advised. However, for the few women with severe anemia who do not respond to iron therapy due to dull erythropoiesis due to infection and/or inflammation, some hematologists consider recombinant human erythropoietin to be an alternative to transfusion.

Regarding the second objective, there are no universally accepted guidelines for the replacement of blood components in patients with obstetric bleeding; recommendations are usually based on expert opinion, as there is no strong evidence from randomized trials, and these opinions are often extrapolated from data from studies in trauma patients, that is, a 1:1:1 replacement; in this case, our suggestion is to administer a packet of platelet apheresis only if the platelet count is less than 50,000/mm^3 [34, 35].

To achieve the objectives of hemostasis and prevention of coagulopathy, it is recommended that you try to raise the level of fibrinogen to a value >300 mg/dl in those situations in which there is active bleeding and in which resuscitation is still being performed, given the highest level of normal basal fibrinogen in pregnancy; however, if we face a controlled bleeding, a fibrinogen value greater than 200 mg/dl will be the objective; the correction of fibrinogen deficiency can be done by using fresh frozen plasma, cryoprecipitate, and fibrinogen concentrates. It is important to emphasize that critically low levels of fibrinogen cannot return to normal using only fresh frozen plasma, without the use of cryoprecipitate or fibrinogen concentrates, since their irrational use only increases the risk of fluid overload and transfusion complications because they only contain a small concentration of fibrinogen in a large volume [35].

Cryoprecipitate is an option for correcting fibrinogen deficiency, but it also contains other clotting factors (VIII, XIII, von Willebrand). The dose depends on the measured and target fibrinogen levels. A reasonable approach is 30 units for fibrinogen <50, 20 units for fibrinogen <100, and 10 units for fibrinogen from 100 to 200. The advantages of cryoprecipitate are that large amounts of fibrinogen can be administered in a low-volume and that it is a low-cost product, and its disadvantages are that it takes time to thaw and prepare for transfusion and that it carries a risk of transmissible infections, since it is a pooled blood product that has not undergone any pathogen inactivation procedure [29, 30].

Another option for correction is fibrinogen concentrate containing approximately 1000 mg of fibrinogen. Usually given alone, it can be used in combination with cryoprecipitate; it is especially useful when fibrinogen levels are critically low (i.e., <100 mg/dl) [36].

Three-factor (II, IX, X) and four-factor (II, VII, IX, X) prothrombin complex concentrates (II, IX, X) are available and have been suggested as an alternative to fresh frozen plasma. The perceived advantages are a reduced risk of volume overload, without the need for thawing or blood typing, and a reduced risk of transfusion-related acute lung injury and allergic reactions. The disadvantages include a very high cost and an increased risk of thrombosis [37].

Recombinant human activated factor VII has been successfully used to control intractable bleeding associated with uterine atony, placenta acreta, or uterine rupture; although this therapy appears to show promise for patients with bleeding refractory to standard therapy, medication is very expensive, and some studies have reported failure in 50% of patients and a possible increase in thrombotic events. Doses range from 16.7 to 120 mcg/kg in a single bolus injection for a few minutes, and repeat the dose every two hours until hemostasis is achieved, usually controlling bleeding within 10 to 40 minutes of the first dose [38].

We additionally recommend:

Maintain oxygenation: Oxygen saturation should be maintained at >95% by administering oxygen (10 to 15 l/minute) through a face mask; if the objective is not achieved, the need for tracheal intubation and mechanical ventilation should be assessed [26, 39].

Avoid hypothermia and **acidosis:** Blood fluids and components must be normothermic to avoid hypothermia, which has been linked to coagulopathy in traumatized patients.

Warming devices (blankets, devices to heat all intravenous fluids, insulating water mattresses, and/or upper and lower body forced-air heating devices) should be used to maintain normothermia (temperature ≥ 35.5°C), since hypothermia results in sympathetic stimulation with increased myocardial oxygen consumption, particularly if chills occur, which can lead to myocardial ischemia. Other adverse consequences of hypothermia include sepsis, coagulopathy, decreased platelet function, and increased mortality [40].

The combination of hypothermia and acidosis increases the risk of clinically significant bleeding despite adequate replacement of blood, plasma, and platelets [26, 40].

In addition, in any mass transfusion situation in which multiple units of blood are rapidly transfused, calcium and potassium should be monitored, with timely treatment of abnormalities. The most common electrolyte abnormalities are low levels of ionized calcium and hyperkalemia. Both disorders, if severe, can lead to cardiac arrest or significantly depressed heart function that prevents optimal resuscitation.

Ionized calcium: Ionized calcium should be measured at baseline and then every 15 to 30 minutes during a massive transfusion and then every hour for the next few hours after transfusions have stopped due to possible hypercalcemia and rebound hypokalemia.

An ionized calcium level < 1 mmol/L (normal 1.1 to 1.3 mmol/L) disrupts clotting and puts the patient at risk of cardiac arrest. Emergency replacement can be achieved by infusion of 1 gram of calcium chloride over two to five minutes through a central line; alternatively, 1 to 2 grams of calcium gluconate can be empirically infused intravenously for two to three minutes for every four units of red blood cells transfused. Hypocalcemia has a linear relationship, a low concentration correlates with a lower concentration of fibrinogen, and a higher likelihood of developing severe acidosis and a lower platelet count.

Potassium: Hyperkalemia can result from rapid transfusion of multiple red blood cell units, especially if they are older units and if they were transfused at a high infusion rate. When an urgent reduction in K+ is needed, a commonly used regimen for delivering insulin and glucose is 10 to 20 units of regular insulin in 500 mL of 10% dextrose, administered intravenously over 60 minutes.

10. Conclusions

Worldwide, every minute, a woman dies due to complications during pregnancy, obstetric hemorrhage being the leading cause; however, most of these deaths are preventable. Hypovolemic shock is the main consequence of obstetric hemorrhage [2, 3].

Patient blood management (PBM) consists of the timely application of evidence-based medical and surgical procedures aimed at maintaining hemoglobin concentration, optimizing hemostasis, and minimizing blood loss to improve patient outcome, considering various strategies to reach the main goal, including transfusional, non-transfusional, and surgical measures.

Despite of the hemodilution, the rheological changes ensure enough oxygen delivery, better placental perfusion, and less risk for thrombosis, despite the bleeding that occurs with childbirth, to improve these objectives being the main outcome of the first pillar [5, 6]. Anemia treatment has the potential to improve outcomes for affected women and their fetuses and neonates and minimize the illness burden and cost due to this common disease [9].

After optimizing the volume of bleeding, the second pillar of management consists of minimizing blood loss, for which its necessary to identify the forecast of surgical bleeding; adequate management of antiplatelet agents and anticoagulants; optimal anesthetic techniques to minimize bleeding; monitoring of the bleeding and coagulopathy; and devising an anesthetic plan.

Apart from the identification and appropriate action in each phase of obstetric hemorrhage, another fundamental pillar in the management of severe primary obstetric hemorrhage is the assessment with laboratory tests that include: blood biometrics, fibrinogen, coagulation studies, and lactate and base deficit (arterial blood gases) as they are tools to evaluate systemic tissue perfusion and are called **"optimal laboratory."**

The objectives in the patient after obstetric hemorrhage are: [26].

- Hemoglobin>7.5 g/dL
- Platelets >50,000/mm^3
- Fibrinogen >200 mg/dL
- Prothrombin time less than 1.5 times the control value.

Author details

Pablo Santillán Roldan[1], Andrés Cepeda Mora[2], Pablo Armas Cruz[3]*, Andres Sarmiento Benavides[3], María Victoria Iturralde Arcos[3], Juan Carlos Jacome Sayay[3], Elisa Aucapiña Chocho[4] and María Isabel Jara Jimbo[4]

1 Obstetric Anesthesiologist at Clínica Atlas, Quito, Ecuador

2 Anesthesiologist and Medical Director of Clínica Atlas, Quito, Ecuador

3 Anesthesiologist at Clínica Atlas, Quito, Ecuador

4 UDLA, Quito, Ecuador

*Address all correspondence to: pablo.armas27@hotmail.com

References

[1] Main EK, McCain CL, Morton CH, Holtby S, Lawton ES. Pregnancy-related mortality in California: causes, characteristics, and improvement opportunities. Obstetrics and Gynecology. 2015;**125**(4):938-947. Available from: https://pubmed.ncbi.nlm.nih.gov/25751214/

[2] Shields LE, Wiesner S, Klein C, Pelletreau B, Hedriana HL. Use of maternal early warning trigger tool reduces maternal morbidity. American Journal of Obstetrics and Gynecology. 2016;**214**(4):527.e1-527.e6. Available from: https://pubmed.ncbi.nlm.nih.gov/26924745/

[3] Anderson JM, Etches D. Prevention and management of postpartum haemorrhage. BJOG. 2022;**124**(5):e106-e1049. Available from: https://onlinelibrary.wiley.com/doi/full/10.1111/1471-0528.14178

[4] WHO recommendations for the prevention and treatment of postpartum haemorrhage. [cited 2022 Dec 5]; Available from: www.who.int/maternal_child_adolescent

[5] Chestnut D et al. Chestnut's Obstetric Anesthesia Principles and Practice. Sixth ed. Elsevier Health; 2019. p. 1324

[6] Kramer MS, Berg C, Abenhaim H, Dahhou M, Rouleau J, Mehrabadi A, et al. Incidence, risk factors, and temporal trends in severe postpartum hemorrhage. American Journal of Obstetrics and Gynecology. 2013;**209**(5):449.e1-449.e7

[7] Bateman BT, Berman MF, Riley LE, Leffert LR. The epidemiology of postpartum hemorrhage in a large, nationwide sample of deliveries. Anesthesia Analgesia. 2010;**110**(5):1368-1373. Available from: https://pubmed.ncbi.nlm.nih.gov/20237047/

[8] Smith C, Teng F, Branch E, Chu S, Joseph KS. Maternal and perinatal morbidity and mortality associated with Anemia in pregnancy. Obstetrics and Gynecology. 2019;**134**(6):1234-1244

[9] PROTOCOLO01_OPTIMIZACION_HB_CIR_PROGRAMADA

[10] WHO recommendations on antenatal care for a positive pregnancy experience.

[11] Carvajal JA, Ramos I, Kusanovic JP, Escobar MF. Damage-control resuscitation in obstetrics. Journal of Maternal-Fetal and Neonatal Medicine. 2022;**35**:785-798

[12] Surbek D, Vial Y, Girard T, Breymann C, Bencaiova GA, Baud D, et al. Patient blood management (PBM) in pregnancy and childbirth: Literature review and expert opinion. Archives of Gynecology and Obstetrics. 2020;**301**:627-641

[13] National Health and Medical Research Council, National Blood Authority (Australia). Patient blood management guidelines. Obstetrics and maternity. 2015;**5**:130

[14] Tibi P, McClure RS, Huang J, Baker RA, Fitzgerald D, Mazer CD, et al. STS/SCA/AmSECT/SABM update to the clinical practice guidelines on patient blood management. Annals of Thoracic Surgery. 2021;**112**(3):981-1004

[15] Hidalgo Martínez F, Cerdán Rodríguez G. Capítulo 13 - Administración de fármacos prohemostáticos: antifibrinolíticos. 2019.

[16] Clevenger B, Mallett S, Klein AA, Richards T. Patient blood management to reduce surgical risk. British Journal of Surgery. 2015;**102**:1325-1337

[17] Augusto PCÁ. MANEJO HEMÁTICO DEL PACIENTE. Mexico; 2020. Available from: http://www.cenetec

[18] Muñoz M, Stensballe J, Ducloy-Bouthors AS, Bonnet MP, de Robertis E, Fornet I, et al. Patient blood management in obstetrics: Prevention and treatment of postpartum haemorrhage. A NATA consensus statement: A multidisciplinary consensus statement. Blood Transfusion. 2019;**17**(2):112-136

[19] Stanworth SJ, Dowling K, Curry N, Doughty H, Hunt BJ, Fraser L, et al. Haematological management of major haemorrhage: A British Society for Haematology guideline. British Journal of Haematology. 2022;**198**(4):654-667

[20] Moreno-Carrillo A, Pulido-Arenas J, Bejarano-Zuleta A, Moreno Carrillo A. Concentrados de complejo protrombinico en el servicio de urgencias. Medicina Interna de México. 2014;**30**:56-63. Available from: www.nietoeditores.com.mx

[21] Ekelund K, Hanke G, Stensballe J, Wikkelsøe A, Albrechtsen CK, Afshari A. Hemostatic resuscitation in postpartum hemorrhage - a supplement to surgery. Acta Obstetricia et Gynecologica Scandinavica. 2015;**94, 2015**:680-692

[22] Luo Y, Ma C, Yu Y. Application of fresh frozen plasma transfusion in the management of excessive warfarin-associated anticoagulation. Blood Science. 2022;**4**(2):57-64

[23] Iglesias PP, Koller Bernhard T, María Gómez-Caro A. Capítulo 11 - Administración de componentes sanguíneos prohemostáticos: fibrinógeno y crioprecipitados. 2019

[24] Hofer S, Schlimp CJ, Casu S, Grouzi E. Management of coagulopathy in bleeding patients. Journal of Clinical Medicine. 2022;**11**:1-17

[25] Hidalgo Martínez F, Aldecoa Á-SC. Capítulo 14 - Hemorragia aguda grave y transfusión masiva. Medicina transfusional perioperatoria. 2019;**2019**

[26] Roberto. "HEMORRAGIA POSTPARTO"

[27] McDonnell NJ, Browning R. How to replace fibrinogen in postpartum haemorrhage situations? (Hint: Don't use FFP!). International Journal of Obstetrics and Anesthesia. 2022;**33**:4-7. Available from: https://pubmed.ncbi.nlm.nih.gov/29017741/

[28] Charbit B, Mandelbrot L, Samain E, Baron G, Haddaoui B, Keita H, et al. The decrease of fibrinogen is an early predictor of the severity of postpartum hemorrhage. Journal of Thrombosis and Hemostasis. 2022;**5**(2):266-273. Available from: https://pubmed.ncbi.nlm.nih.gov/17087729/

[29] Cortet M, Deneux-Tharaux C, Dupont C, Colin C, Rudigoz RC, Bouvier-Colle MH, et al. Association between fibrinogen level and severity of postpartum haemorrhage: Secondary analysis of a prospective trial. British Journal of Anaesthia. 2012;**108**(6):984-989. Available from: https://pubmed.ncbi.nlm.nih.gov/22490316/

[30] Collins PW, Lilley G, Bruynseels D, Laurent DBS, Cannings-John R, Precious E, et al. Fibrin-based clot formation as an early and rapid biomarker for progression of postpartum hemorrhage: A prospective study. Blood. 2014;**124**(11):1727-1736. Available from: https://pubmed.ncbi.nlm.nih.gov/25024304/

[31] van der Bom JG. Viscoelastometric testing, fibrinogen and transfusion during post-partum haemorrhage. British Journal of Anaesthia. 2017;**119**(3):352-353. Available from: https://pubmed.ncbi.nlm.nih.gov/28969322/

[32] Szecsi PB, Jørgensen M, Klajnbard A, Andersen MR, Colov NP, Stender S. Haemostatic reference intervals in pregnancy. Thrombosis and Haemostosis. 2022;**103**(4):718-727. Available from: https://pubmed.ncbi.nlm.nih.gov/20174768/

[33] Fuller AJ, Bucklin B. Blood component therapy in obstetrics. Obstetrics and Gynecology Clinical North America. 2007;**34**(3):443-458. Available from: https://pubmed.ncbi.nlm.nih.gov/17921009/

[34] A mathematical model for fresh frozen plasma transfusion strategies during major trauma resuscitation with ongoing hemorrhage - PubMed [Internet]. [cited 2022 Dec 5]. Available from: https://pubmed.ncbi.nlm.nih.gov/16417053/

[35] Allard S, Green L, Hunt BJ. How we manage the haematological aspects of major obstetric haemorrhage. British Journal of Haematology. 2014;**164**(2):177-188. Available from: https://onlinelibrary.wiley.com/doi/full/10.1111/bjh.12605

[36] Ahmed S, Harrity C, Johnson S, Varadkar S, Mcmorrow S, Fanning R, et al. The efficacy of fibrinogen concentrate compared with cryoprecipitate in major obstetric haemorrhage--an observational study. Transfusion Medical. 2012;**22**(5):344-349. Available from: https://pubmed.ncbi.nlm.nih.gov/22994449/

[37] Nuttall GA, Brost BC, Connis RT, Gessner JS, Harrison CR, Miller RD, et al. Practice guidelines for perioperative blood transfusion and adjuvant therapies: An updated report by the American Society of Anesthesiologists Task Force on Perioperative Blood Transfusion and Adjuvant Therapies. Anesthesiology. 2006;**105**(1):198-208. Available from: https://pubmed.ncbi.nlm.nih.gov/16810012/

[38] Lavigne-Lissalde G, Aya AG, Mercier FJ, Roger-Christoph S, Chauleur C, Morau E, et al. Recombinant human FVIIa for reducing the need for invasive second-line therapies in severe refractory postpartum hemorrhage: a multicenter, randomized, open controlled trial. Journal of Thrombosis and Haemostosis. 2015;**13**(4):520-529. Available from: https://pubmed.ncbi.nlm.nih.gov/25594352/

[39] Likis FE, Sathe NA, Morgans AK, Hartmann KE, Young JL, Carlson-Bremer D, et al. Management of Postpartum Hemorrhage. 2015 [cited 2022 Dec 5]. Available from: https://www.ncbi.nlm.nih.gov/books/NBK294465/

[40] Ferrara A, MacArthur JD, Wright HK, Modlin IM, McMillen MA. Hypothermia and acidosis worsen coagulopathy in the patient requiring massive transfusion. American Journal of Surgery. 1990;**160**(5):515-518. Available from: https://pubmed.ncbi.nlm.nih.gov/2240386/